CBT

A Clinician's Guide to Using the Five Areas Approach

Dr Chris Williams
Marie Chellingsworth

CBT

A Clinician's Guide to Using the Five Areas Approach

Dr Chris Williams BSc (Hons) MBChB MMedSc MD FRCPsych
BABCP Accredited CBT practitioner
Professor of Psychosocial Psychiatry and Honorary Consultant Psychiatrist, Section of Psychological Medicine, Faculty of Medicine, University of Glasgow, UK

Marie Chellingsworth RMN Dip Nursing BSc (Hons)
Course Director (IAPT) and Senior Lecturer in Psychological Therapies, Faculty of Medicine and Health Sciences, School of Nursing, Midwifery and Physiotherapy, University of Nottingham, and Senior Fellow of the Institute of Mental Health, Nottingham, UK

Helping you to help yourself
www.livinglifetothefull.com (www.llttf.com)
www.livinglifetothefullinteractive.com (www.llttfi.com)
www.fiveareas.com
www.fiveareasonline.com
www.fiveareastraining.com

CRC Press
Taylor & Francis Group
Boca Raton London New York

CRC Press is an imprint of the
Taylor & Francis Group, an **informa** business

CRC Press
Taylor & Francis Group
6000 Broken Sound Parkway NW, Suite 300
Boca Raton, FL 33487-2742

First issued in hardback 2017

Version Date: 20170124

ISBN-13: 978-0-340-99129-9 (pbk)
ISBN-13: 978-1-138-44533-8 (hbk)

Visit the Taylor & Francis Web site at
http://www.taylorandfrancis.com

and the CRC Press Web site at
http://www.crcpress.com

Accessing the worksheets

Electronic (PDF) versions of the worksheet handouts in this book and many more are available from **www.fiveareas.com**.

PDF versions of the workbooks

Copies of the workbooks and other Five Areas books published by Hodder Arnold are available under licence from the publisher for use on restricted access, password-protected health service computer servers. This allows high-quality copies of the workbooks to be printed off by a defined number of practitioners or patients/clients.

For more information please contact: Jenny Davis, Rights Manager, Hodder Education, 338 Euston Road, London NW1 3BH.
Tel: +44 (0) 20 7873 6286, email: **jenny.davis@hodder.co.uk**

Buying the books in bulk: Bulk copies of the book are available at discounted rates direct from the publisher.

To take advantage of these reduced rates please contact: Jane MacRae, Sales Development Manager, Hodder Education, 338 Euston Road, London NW1 3BH.
Tel: +44 (0) 20 7873 6146, email: **jane.macrae@hodder.co.uk**

Translations, large print and screen-reader versions

For **translation requests** please contact the publisher.

Licensed versions of this book and large print versions online are available in screen-reader format for those with visual problems at **www.fiveareasonline.com.**

Cartoon illustrations

Cartoon illustrations are by Keith Chan and are available for clinical use from **www.fiveareas.com.**

Contents

Introduction ix

Part 1 Getting to know the Five Areas approach

Chapter 1: Why is there a need for accessible forms of cognitive behavioural therapy? 2

Chapter 2: Key elements of the Five Areas model 12

Part 2 Using the Five Areas approach

Clinical assessment and selling the model

Chapter 3: Completing a collaborative Five Areas assessment 36

Chapter 4: Using the Five Areas assessment to understand why the person feels as they do 58

Supporting and reviewing progress

Chapter 5: Setting goals and monitoring progress using the Plan, Do, Review model 78

Chapter 6: Offering structured support face to face and by telephone or email 92

Chapter 7: Delivering support in the LLTTF and other classes 110

Part 3 Resources overview

Chapter 8: Five Areas written resources for low mood and stress 128

Chapter 9: Five Areas online, DVD and audio multimedia resources for low mood and stress 148

Part 4 Supervision, training and service implications

Chapter 10: Case management and supervision 158

Chapter 11: Training and supporting practitioners in using the Five Areas approach 169

Part 5 The Five Areas in action

Five Areas model as a first contact assessment tool in an IAPT team in England 189

Five Areas books with GP support 190

Five Areas depression book plus telephone support in Canada 192

Use of the *Overcoming anxiety* book in an IAPT service 194

Little CBT Books delivered by housing workers in England 195

Little CBT Books delivered by social services via telephone and LLTTF classes 197

LLTTF classes delivered in community settings 199

LLTTF classes with university students 201

LLTTF classes in schools 203

Using the Little CBT Books in secondary schools 204

Living Life to the Full free online course (**www.llttf.com**) 206

Living Life to the Full Interactive (**www.llttf.com**) offered across Scotland (pilot service) 208

Overcoming Bulimia Online (**www.overcomingbulimiaonline.com**) delivered in a specialist eating disorders service 210

Overcoming Anorexia Online (**www.overcominganorexiaonline.com**) delivered in a specialist eating disorders clinic 212

Self-help clinic in a primary care mental health team 214

Part 6 Supporter scripts and resources 217

Introduction

We hope you tear up this book ...

Tear it up? Well, yes, because it's a book to be used. It contains a wealth of practical learning from research and clinical delivery, and is based on feedback from clinicians, voluntary sector colleagues and people who have used the approach in practice. From this we have distilled a range of practical 'how to' learning points that address the key questions that are asked again and again:

- Who can use the cognitive behavioural therapy (CBT) approach?
- How do you best introduce and support the resources in everyday clinical work?
- What if someone feels stuck?
- How do you decide which resource is the most helpful?
- What if you only have limited time?

and more...

Who is this book for?

These resources are aimed at:

- Health, social and voluntary sector workers wanting to gain an overview of the Five Areas CBT approach and specific skills on how to assess, introduce and support people in using the various Five Areas resources.
- Managers and commissioners planning to redesign their services to include a range of high and low intensity approaches.

Why use the Five Areas approach?

Mental health problems are common and distressing. Words used in formal clinical diagnoses of depression and anxiety such as 'mild' and 'moderate' to describe severity fail to do justice to just how nasty low mood and anxiety are for the person, their family and friends. Fortunately, effective treatments exist – and these include both medication, such as antidepressants, and also psychotherapeutic approaches.

Evidence-based reviews confirm that the CBT approach has the widest application across mental and physical health disorders. However, the biggest current challenge is how to provide wide access to the CBT approach. Currently, for many, access to CBT delivered by specialists is still restricted. This restriction is not only because of a lack of specialised practitioners but also other issues that restrict use, including the need for patients to travel, attend during normal working hours and then have to spend some of their already flagging mental energy learning the complex language used in CBT. A key issue in CBT (as indicated by initials such as CBT) is therefore how to communicate the model clearly without the use of jargon.

This book highlights two possible solutions:

- A usable, pragmatic and flexible 'translation' of CBT into a more accessible and everyday language.
- The need to offer CBT interventions in all sorts of sizes and shapes so that people can work on their problems in ways that they want and that fit their lives.

This book is therefore designed to help you to help people:

- Learn important information about how mental and physical health problems can affect their life.
- Work out why they are feeling as they do.
- Provide the right sort of support and tools they need to start and keep working on overcoming their problems.

Linked online resources

Various free resources are available online to support practitioners:

- An online training course covering the key elements of how to introduce, support and review progress of those using the Five Areas approach. This is available in the practitioner area of **www.llttf.com**. Simply register as a practitioner to access these.
- Regular newsletters with hints and tips and updates on resources.

A second dedicated website for practitioner training is in development at **www.fiveareastraining.com**.

Local training and support

Training from experienced Five Areas trainers can be arranged with courses ranging from one to three days and covering the use of any of the Five Areas resources. Contact **training@fiveareas.com** for further information.

A note about copyright

Acknowledgements and dedication

The illustrations in the workbooks have been produced by Keith Chan, **kchan75@hotmail.com**. Copies are available at **www.fiveareas.com** as a separate download for clinical use.

Finally, we wish to thank Alison, Hannah and Andrew Williams and John Chellingsworth, who have supported us during the writing of this book.

Dedicated to the memory of Bridget Chellingsworth.

Dr Chris Williams Ms Marie Chellingsworth

August 2010

PART 1

Getting to know the Five Areas approach

Chapter 1

Why is there a need for accessible forms of cognitive behavioural therapy?

What you will learn

In this chapter you will learn about:

- Why CBT is increasingly recommended in national treatment guidelines.
- The need for patients to receive CBT in accessible ways.
- The need for practitioners to be taught CBT in accessible ways.
- How to produce CBT resources that are accessible and available in different sizes and shapes.
- The matched care approach.

Introduction

CBT stands for cognitive behavioural therapy. Although this is a convenient label to describe a general approach, it is perhaps best to think of CBT as a range of different treatment models, addressing a range of different disorders, which has at its heart the proposition that **how a person thinks affects how they feel and alters what they do**. This chapter will describe what CBT is and provide a brief review of its evolution to date, and explain why we feel it is inevitable that services will increasingly offer CBT in all sorts of sizes and shapes.

The development of CBT

Cognitive behavioural therapy was first described by Professor Aaron Beck in the USA during the early 1950s. He and another pioneer, Professor Albert Ellis, laid the foundation for the subsequent growth of CBT approaches. In the UK, the first training courses began only in the late 1970s, and the growth in CBT from then on was linked to two main factors:

- A growing evidence base: CBT has always seen itself a therapy based on empirical science. Positive outcome studies have led it to be recommended by national treatment guidelines such as those produced by the National Institute for Health and Clinical Excellence (NICE) in England and the Scottish Intercollegiate Guidelines Network (SIGN) in Scotland.

- The writing of the seminal textbook *Cognitive therapy for depression* (Beck *et al.*, 1979): Prior to the publication of this book, CBT was largely taught by a core group of interested practitioners. This book, however, manualised/operationalised CBT, and allowed it to be disseminated far more widely – and far more quickly.

The rapid development of CBT models is also exemplified by the growing range of disorders for which CBT has an evidence base.

The evidence base for CBT

Cognitive behavioural therapy has the widest range and greatest depth of evidence supporting its effectiveness compared with any other form of psychotherapy. Initially CBT was developed for psychosis (Beck 1952), and then depression (Beck et al., 1979), but this quickly expanded to include disorders such as anxiety disorders, personality disorders, alcohol and substance misuse, bipolar disorder, psychosis/schizophrenia, post-traumatic stress disorder, bulimia nervosa, and a range of physical (e.g. pain, fatigue, arthritis and more) and wider interventions (e.g. back-to-work initiatives and for compliance/adherence to medication). There is therefore a growing list of recommendations for CBT.

Importantly, CBT has **not** been shown to be an effective intervention for some disorders, such as anorexia nervosa, so it is not to be assumed automatically that CBT is the answer to every possible area of distress or other problems.

Challenges to the roll out of CBT

Between the 1980s and 1990s there was a rapid increase in the development of specialist CBT units, and a growing cohort of specialist practitioners from various professional backgrounds who had received training in CBT. By the end of the 1990s most non-CBT practitioners had a fairly clear idea of what a referral 'for CBT' would entail. At that time, being referred for a course of CBT meant that the patient would see an expert practitioner, often accredited as a CBT, CT or BT (cognitive therapy or behaviour therapy) practitioner by, for example, the lead body for CBT in the UK – the British Association for Behavioural and Cognitive Psychotherapies (**www.babcp.com**). The patient would have an initial assessment, and if found to have an appropriate clinical problem for which CBT had an evidence base, they would be offered a 'course' of CBT. This traditionally lasted between 12 and 20 sessions, with each session lasting about an hour.

However, the rise in awareness of the benefits of CBT led to a rapidly increasing referral rate, which resulted in a significant mismatch between demand and supply. Consequently, far more people were referred for treatment than could possibly be seen within existing services. The result was waiting lists and a situation where services with waiting lists opted to respond to this by tightening their entry criteria for CBT.

The use of selection criteria that emphasised factors such as chronicity and severity led to a focus on the delivery of services predominantly for the most complex and chronic cases. This led to a paradox where those people who could potentially benefit the most from CBT (i.e. those with mild to moderately severe depression, anxiety and panic) were least likely to be offered it and patients whose conditions were least responsive to CBT receiving it – thereby exacerbating the issue of waiting lists. As a result, there quickly developed a situation where there were strong inequalities in terms of access to CBT across the UK.

The case for delivering both low and high intensity CBT

The lack of access and capacity in services and the growing resultant inequalities was the focus of a much quoted paper by Lovell and Richards (2000) called Maple (Multiple Access Points and Levels of Entry), which acted as a catalyst for service redesign. Lovell and Richards argued that although there was an evidence base for delivering CBT in the traditional way (12–20 one-hour sessions), there was also a growing evidence base that CBT could be offered in a range of other ways. Later to be described as low intensity CBT (LI), their paper described two additional ways (levels of entry) that CBT could be offered:

- Wider access approaches, such as CBT self-help and group treatments.
- The delivery of key components of CBT such as *progressive exposure and response prevention* for anxiety, and *behavioural activation* for depression. Lovell and Richards pointed to the so-called dismantling studies that had compared specific aspects of the CBT model, such as behavioural activation, with cognitive interventions alone, and also with the full cognitive and behavioural therapy interventions combined. These studies confirmed (and continue to confirm) that patients can equally benefit from working on behavioural aspects of care alone as they can when offered the (longer) full CBT model. Lovell and Richards therefore argued that patients should typically be offered more focused, and shorter, interventions before being offered the full, specialist CBT model. Their paper also pointed the way to telephone-delivered support and the differentiation of low and high intensity working.

There has followed in the past 10 years a revolution in the development of a wide range of so-called low intensity interventions. Low intensity working refers to reduced practitioner time to support the intervention. So, for example, much of the CBT may be delivered via a self-help package. Sessions tend to be shorter in terms of time (10–30 minutes) and length (often 3–10 support sessions). This contrasts with high intensity CBT (HI) with its 12–20+ longer sessions (typically one hour).

The evidence base for low intensity working

The evidence base for delivering low intensity working has progressively strengthened over the past 10 years. There are now numerous systematic reviews and meta-analyses examining the effectiveness of CBT self-help for example. A key review by Gellatly *et al.* (2007) brings together the evidence base for CBT self-help, and summarises not just the evidence base for this but also how best to support the use of CBT self-help for depression. Gellatly and colleagues found that:

- CBT self-help resources are far more effective than psychoeducational resources for the treatment of depression.
- The addition of support is crucial and improves outcomes significantly.
- There is no difference between computer-based and written ways of delivering CBT self-help. In other words the issue is one of how the patient wants to learn.

CBT self-help is now recommended as a first step for care for mild to moderate depression in recent practice guidelines such as those produced by NICE (2009) and SIGN (2010), where it has been judged to have category A high quality supporting evidence.

Box 1.1 Low intensity (reproduced with permission from Bennett-Levy *et al.*, 2010)

The primary purpose of low intensity CBT interventions is to increase access to evidence-based psychological therapies in order to enhance mental health and wellbeing on a community-wide basis, using the minimum level of intervention necessary to create the maximum gain. Low intensity CBT interventions have been mainly developed in the context of patients with mild to moderate psychological disorders, enabling high intensity CBT to be reserved for patients with more severe disorders. Therefore, compared with high intensity CBT, low intensity interventions:

- Reduce the amount of time the practitioner is in contact with individual patients – whether this is reduced through seeing more than one patient at the same time (i.e. group CBT); *or* seeing them for fewer/shorter sessions (i.e. advice clinics); *or* supporting their use of self-help materials (i.e. self-help books, internet-based CBT interventions); *or* facilitating their engagement with community and voluntary resources *and/or*
- Use practitioners specifically trained to deliver low intensity CBT, who may not have formal health professional or high-intensity CBT qualifications, e.g. paraprofessionals, peer supporters, voluntary sector *and/or*
- Use CBT resources whose content is often less intense (self-paced, own time, bite-size pieces) *and/or*
- Provide more rapid access to early intervention and preventive CBT programmes.

Low intensity CBT interventions aim to communicate key CBT principles in accessible ways, and to deliver content in a variety of flexible forms – face-to-face, email, groups, phone-based – which maximise the opportunity for patient choice. Typically, low intensity CBT interventions are simple and brief. They focus on the use of CBT self-help materials and techniques, emphasise the value of between-session homework, and assess, monitor and evaluate progress as an intrinsic part of the intervention. The content may constitute a treatment intervention in itself (e.g. behavioural activation, internet-based therapy, guided CBT), may support or promote an intervention (e.g. motivational enhancement, '10 minute CBT' GP consultations, advice clinics), or may be preventive of treatment interventions (preventive/educational programmes).

Compared with traditional services for patients with mental health problems, low intensity CBT interventions increase:

- Access and/or speed of access to treatment
- The total number of people who can access evidence-based treatments
- Service flexibility, responsiveness and capacity
- Patient choice
- Cost-effectiveness of services.

Why CBT self-help is an effective way of delivering CBT

However offered, CBT is fundamentally a self-help form of psychotherapy: it aims to help people become their own therapist; it focuses on helping people work out why they feel as they do; and it teaches key (evidence-based, tried and trusted) interventions to help overcome problems (using problem-solving approaches), change extreme and unhelpful thinking, and alter behaviour to helpfully boost how the person feels.

New ways of working

Based on the growing evidence base, and the problem of waiting lists for CBT, a number of pilot interventions have been trialled, which have then led on to far larger roll-out programmes. In Scotland the Doing Well by People with Depression Programme (**www.scotland.gov.uk/Publications/2005/07/2994711/47119**) and the WISH Programme (widening access to self-help, e.g. **www.dascot.org/services/livinglifetothefull/index.html#llttfi**) have piloted ways of introducing low intensity working in order to improve the capacity of services to provide evidence-based treatments. WISH is currently offering training to practitioners working in three large health board areas in Scotland in how to use the Five Areas CBT model and is described in more detail on pages 206–208 in Part 5.

In England, experience at the initial pilot sites in Newham and Doncaster has led to the development of the large Increasing Access to Psychological Therapies (IAPT) programme (**www.iapt.nhs.uk**). This has further led to a renewed focus on the delivery of low and high intensity CBT and on clarifying the differences between these two approaches. Numerous local teams consisting of low and high intensity workers are radically altering how quickly people can access CBT near to where they live, or from their own homes by telephone.

Although the case for low intensity working seems clear, it has proved quite a challenge developing models of training, supervision and delivery that are accessible and usable by patients and practitioners and which can be incorporated into existing and new ways of working (**www.newwaysofworking.org.uk**). One important issue when considering how to introduce a range of CBT self-help resources into services is the language used to communicate the CBT model.

Issues of language: CBT self-help or guided CBT?

Language matters. It affects how treatments are perceived – especially when those treatments are novel and not necessarily understood by the patient. So, for example, in services when patients are given the choice of computerised CBT (cCBT) or book-based CBT self-help (sometimes called *bibliotherapy*), the majority choose books. A recent study investigated whether individuals would opt to use cCBT. It found that only a minority would initially choose to use cCBT if depressed; however, the proportion willing to use the cCBT resource increased greatly when the person was allowed to actually see the resources (Mitchell and Gordon 2007). This raises three important points:

- **Information may need to be given to patients about the clinical service and the support options available**. For example, using information sheets or informational DVDs or through providing hands-on experience (e.g. see excerpts from some of the books, DVD, cCBT resources) so that decisions are based on informed choice. For example, a sample session from **www.llttfi.com** is available at **www.livinglifetothefullinteractive.co.uk/Portals/0/LLTTFDemo/LLTTFiDemo.html**. However, too much choice can also be confusing. This means that when providing information it is not always helpful to provide a vast menu of intervention options. Instead one of the benefits of assessment is also to provide people with an informed range of *treatment recommendations* that are appropriate for them. This is discussed in more detail in Chapters 3–5.

- **People like to work in difference ways**. What matters is choosing a mode of working that is attractive and relevant to them.
- **Language matters**. Terms such as 'computerised' or even 'self-help' raise certain expectations of what will be offered. Such expectations may be inaccurate or unhelpful. For example, the term 'self-help' implies that the patient works on their own to address their problems. This is often the last thing the patient wants when they have finally plucked up courage to seek help. We much prefer a term introduced by Dr Hendrik Hinrichsen, lead at the Wimbledon and Morton IAPT team in London, which is *guided CBT*. This highlights two key aspects of what is being offered: first, that the intervention is based on CBT; and second, that it is not just handed out or 'prescribed' but it is used within the context of a supportive relationship.

Challenges to the delivery of guided CBT and high intensity CBT

In many ways the arguments for low intensity working seem clear. However, there are some practical problems that are shared by both high and low intensity CBT working.

The traditional language of CBT is complex and difficult to communicate

Many practitioners when first exposed to CBT training spend significant time learning the traditional language of CBT. This includes complex technical terms such as cognitive errors, schemas, dichotomous thinking and negative automatic thoughts. These are terms that are very helpful in scientific evaluations of how thinking alters during therapy, but are not easily understood by lay people. It is asking a lot of patients with mental health problems, however mild or severe, to learn the traditional language of CBT before they can start working with the practitioner. Workers in low intensity and high intensity CBT know this and adjust for it in one-to-one care. However, many widely used CBT self-help books utilise complex language and styles that make the books overwhelming and hard to read for many.

Reading age is the age at which 50% of a population of that age can readily understand the content of a target publication. It is usually evaluated using complex mathematical equations incorporating factors such as sentence, word and paragraph length. Different reading scales exist, and some also calculate the reading difficulty by comparing the words used against lists of commonly used, and also low frequency/more complex words. Typically practitioners would wish someone to read materials that have a reading age of one to two years less than their actual reading ability so that they can read the resource with some ease. So, a resource for someone with a reading age of 14–15+ should have a reading age of between 12–13. For example, in a summary of reading ages of a range of commonly recommended CBT self-help resources Martinez *et al.* (2008) found that *Overcoming Depression and Low Mood: The Five Areas Approach* had the lowest reading age, at 12.6 years. None of the other widely used existing CBT self-help resources achieved this level.

To put this in context, the reading age of the *Scottish Sun* is 12–13 years, and that of *The Financial Times* and *Guardian* newspapers is around 17 (Martinez *et al.*, 2008). At the same time, around 16 per cent of people struggle in the UK to read at reading age 11. Unfortunately, the reading age of the traditional CBT model is over 17 (Williams and Garland 2002).

CBT self-help resources often show poor design

A lot has been written about how to produce patient information materials that are accessible, designed for a particular population, and are easily used. For example:

- Use of fonts such as Arial.
- A font size that is >10, preferably 12.
- Shorter sentences in the active tense (Jack kicked the ball) rather than passive (the ball was kicked by Jack), which is more difficult to understand.
- White space between paragraphs and topics, so as to chunk information and break text up into paragraphs.
- Case examples (e.g. examples of people experiencing the same problem) are particularly popular with people using self-help resources.
- The use of the words *I*, *you* and *we* can affect how people judge a resource as being personal and engaging or as a purely factual report.
- Encouraging the reader to interact with the materials as they read them. So, incorporating questions and worksheets can be a helpful way of helping people to immediately try and test out in their own lives what they are reading.
- Illustrations can not only be helpful but also can sometimes put people off. For example, it can be better to avoid consistent age, gender or race case examples unless a resource is specifically aimed at a particular group.

The ability of a self-help book to communicate and establish a therapeutic relationship may also predict its effectiveness (Richardson *et al.*, 2008).

Expert practitioners do not believe low intensity working is as 'good' as high intensity working

Several surveys have shown that high intensity workers often use CBT self-help resources. Yet they often tend to judge such low intensity ways of working as being less effective than high intensity working (Whitfield and Williams, 2004). This conflicts with results of most studies that have confirmed equivalence of outcome (Cuijpers *et al.*, 2010). In addition, non-attendance and early drop out rates for high intensity work do not suggest that it is a method of working which is significantly more attractive and engaging (Williams and Martinez, 2008). What is probably true is that patients prefer to work in different ways. Some will prefer high intensity working and others low intensity working. Some will run a mile before wanting to attend one-hour high intensity sessions, whereas for others even telephone support may seem too much and they may prefer email support. The key here is engaging patients in ways they feel able to commit to – and to work together from there.

Models of training focusing on low intensity work have not until recently existed

The first UK-based university-accredited low intensity CBT course was the SPIRIT (Structured Psychosocial InteRventions) course based at Glasgow Caledonian University. A range of other low intensity courses have now also been developed as part of the IAPT courses in England, and in Scotland the universities of Dundee/Stirling offer an MSc in psychological therapy in primary care. Linked to this, there have been until recently very few training resources that have focused on low intensity working. This is slowly changing with the current book, and other books such as Bennett-Levy *et al.* (2010).

Supervision models have not been appropriate for low intensity working

The far larger caseloads held by low intensity workers (which can be up to 60 patients at one time – compared with up to 20 for high intensity workers) have forced the development of appropriate new ways of working requiring low intensity supervision models. Indeed, in the IAPT approach the term *supervision* is not used at all; instead the term *case management* is used. This approach can include the use of automated online alerts for practitioners and supervisors which automatically flag cases for routine review at set time points, and also when there is evidence of deterioration, drop out and risk (e.g. see **www.pc-mis.co.uk**). The different models are described in Chapter 10.

There is a need for practitioners to be taught CBT in accessible ways

In low intensity working the competencies required for effective working are more focused than those required for high intensity practice. Courses can vary from 38 hours (SPIRIT – see **www.fiveareastraining.com**) for staff who already possess core skills such as knowledge of the professional relationship, ethical working, the need for clinical confidentiality, and how to create NHS records and communicate professionally. Longer courses such as those in the IAPT training in England are delivered over 45 days (25 days within a university setting and 20 days in supervised practice). This includes modules on core safe working and assessment and engagement, CBT self-help and other interventions and how to support them, reaching diverse groups, and looking at employment needs and supervision. These are run as postgraduate certificate courses at institutions certified by IAPT as being approved training providers.

Making CBT accessible: matched care

Matched care implies that the patient is offered the type of intervention they need, delivered in a form they can engage in, and with support that is acceptable and easily used by them. In practice this means that practitioners need to offer an evidence-based intervention that is:

- Usually CBT-based for many (but not all) mental health disorders. Other evidence-based psychotherapies can also, of course, be offered as appropriate.
- Delivered in a form/modality that the patient finds acceptable (e.g. books, computers, DVDs or a focused form of intervention such as behavioural activation).

- Accompanied by the type of (e.g. face-to-face, telephone, email, live chat, videoconferencing or using classes) and amount of support the patient needs (varying the length and frequency of support sessions required, so, for example, CBT self-help can also be offered in longer high intensity settings).

Key practice points

- CBT and CBT self-help approaches are both evidence based treatments.
- Supported CBT self-help is far more effective than unsupported CBT self-help.
- Self-help resources need to be appropriate, accessible and available in a format the patient is happy to use.
- Patients should be supported in ways they can engage in and find effective.
- The term *guided CBT* is a helpful term that can be used in services to describe the introduction of CBT self-help approaches.

References

Beck AT. (1952) Successful outpatient psychotherapy of a chronic schizophrenic with a delusion based on borrowed guilt. *Psychiatry* **15**: 305–12.

Beck AT, Rush AJ, Shaw BF, Emery G. (1979) *Cognitive therapy of depression*. New York: Guilford Press.

Bennett-Levy J, Richards D, Farrand P, Christensen H *et al.* (eds). (2010) *Oxford guide to low intensity CBT interventions* (Oxford Guides in Cognitive Behavioural Therapy). Oxford: Oxford University Press.

Cuijpers P, Donker T, van Straten A, Li J, Anderson, G. (2010) Is guided self-help as effective as face-to-face psychotherapy for depression and anxiety disorders? A systematic review and meta-analysis. *Psychological Medicine*, in press.

Gellatly J, Bower P, Hennessy S, Richards D *et al.* (2007) What makes self-help interventions effective in the management of depressive symptoms? Meta-analysis and meta-regression. *Psychological Medicine* **37**: 1217–28.

Lovell K, Richards D. (2000) Multiple Access Points and Levels of Entry (MAPLE): ensuring choice, accessibility and equity for CBT services. *Behavioural and Cognitive Psychotherapy* **28**: 379–91.

Martinez R, Whitfield G, Dafters R, Williams CJ. (2008) Can people read self-help manuals for depression? A challenge for the stepped care model and book prescription schemes. *Behavioural and Cognitive Psychotherapy* **36**: 89–97.

Mitchell N, Gordon PK. (2007) Attitudes towards computerized CBT for depression amongst a student population. *Behavioural and Cognitive Psychotherapy* **35**: 421–30.

National Institute for Health and Clinical Excellence (NICE). (2009) Depression: Management of depression in primary and secondary care. Clinical guideline 90. London: National Institute for Health and Clinical Excellence.

Richardson R, Richards DA, Barkham MB. (2008) Self-help books for people with depression: a scoping review. *Journal of Mental Health* **17**: 543–52.

Scottish Intercollegiate Guidelines Network (SIGN). (2010) Guideline 114: Non-pharmaceutical treatment of depression in adults: a national clinical guideline. Available at: **www.sign.ac.uk/pdf/sign114.pdf**.

Whitfield G, Williams CJ. (2004) If the evidence is so good why doesn't anyone use them? Current uses of computer-based self-help packages. *Behavioural and Cognitive Psychotherapy* **32**: 57–65.

Williams CJ, Garland A. (2002) A cognitive behavioural therapy assessment model for use in everyday clinical practice. *Advances in Psychiatric Treatment* **8**: 172–9.

Williams CJ, Martinez R. (2008) Increasing access to CBT: stepped care and CBT self-help models in practice. *Behavioural and Cognitive Psychotherapy* **36**: 675–83.

Further reading

Bennett-Levy J, Richards D, Farrand P, Christensen H *et al.* (eds). (2010) *Oxford guide to low intensity CBT interventions* (Oxford Guides in Cognitive Behavioural Therapy). Oxford: Oxford University Press.

Duman M. (2003) *Producing patient information: how to research, develop and produce effective information resources*, 2nd edn. London: King's Fund.

Macleod M, Martinez R, Williams CJ. (2009) Cognitive behaviour therapy self-help: who does it help and what are its drawbacks? *Behavioural and Cognitive Psychotherapy* **37**: 61–72.

Martinez R, Whitfield G, Dafters R, Williams CJ. (2008) Can people read self-help manuals for depression? A challenge for the stepped care model and book prescription schemes. *Behavioural and Cognitive Psychotherapy* **36**: 89–97.

Richards DA, Lovell K, Gilbody S, Gask L *et al.* (2008) Collaborative care for depression in UK primary care: a randomised controlled trial. *Psychological Medicine* **38**: 279–87.

Chapter 2

Key elements of the Five Areas model

What you will learn

In this chapter you will learn about:

- The Five Areas model.
- The language used to describe altered thinking.
- The language used to describe altered behaviour.
- Identifying targets for change.
- The seven-step problem solving approach.
- The Five Areas assessment in low and high intensity settings.
- Systemic assessments using the Five Areas model.
- Online training resources.

Other related chapters are Chapters 3–5.

Introduction

It is well recognised that cognitive behavioural therapy is a helpful approach for making sense of and improving problems in many clinical disorders (Chapter 1). As outlined in Chapter 1, although CBT has many advantages, it also uses a complex and technical language that asks a lot of patients – especially if they have to learn that language before they can start work on the process of change.

This chapter introduces the Five Areas model. The Five Areas model aims to communicate key CBT principles concerning understanding of the problem, and changing thinking and behaviour in a simple and straightforward way to help patients and practitioners alike to make sense of symptoms. Through the use of engaging and everyday language, the approach retains the benefits of CBT in terms of its structure and step-by-step way of helping patients plan changes to their life.

The Five Areas approach

The term 'cognitive behavioural therapy' implies a focus on thoughts (cognitions) and behaviours. In fact CBT examines far more than this and provides a flexible whole person bio-psychosocial assessment. The Five Areas assessment helps to summarise the problems/ symptoms faced by the person in the five key areas of life. The five areas are:

Area 1: The situations faced. This area includes the **people and events** around the person. For some, these may be problematic, causing upset and stress; for others, they will be supportive and helpful. For yet others, there may be a sense of isolation with no-one around them.

Area 2: **Altered thinking**. This can often become extreme and unhelpful – especially during times of distress when a person feels anxious or low.

Area 3: **Altered feelings** (also called moods or emotions).

Area 4: **Altered physical symptoms**, which are often associated with low mood (e.g. low energy and tiredness) or anxiety (e.g. tension and a rapid heart rate) or may be because of a concurrent physical illness (such as diabetes or angina).

Area 5: **Altered behaviour or activity levels**. This includes both the *helpful* things people can do to try to feel better, and the *unhelpful things* they can sometimes do too – which backfire and make them feel even worse, such as drinking too much.

Key Point

As well as identifying problems and difficulties, the Five Areas approach also helps the person recognise what is going well, and what resources they have within or around them that might aid recovery, for example being in a job, having access to financial savings, having a close friend or family member to talk to, or having a child who is loved. It might also include things such as having a sense of humour or having a hobby that is enjoyed – or at least a past history of some of these things that can be reintroduced during treatment.

Completing a Five Areas assessment in low intensity CBT

There are several ways of helping people complete a Five Areas assessment:

- The patient can complete the assessment themselves by going through a self-assessment workbook (such as the *Understanding why you feel as you do* workbook in the *Overcoming Depression and Low Mood* book).
- They could also complete their own interactive Five Areas assessment using an online Five Areas package such as **www.llttfi.com**. Practitioners and patients both can try this now using the free online demo at **www.livinglifetothefullinteractive.co.uk/ Portals/0/LLTTFDemo/LLTTFiDemo.html**.
- Alternatively, a practitioner can lead the initial assessment – and from this generate a Five Areas assessment. This can be done during a short session or series of shorter sessions (e.g. 10–30 minutes), or over a longer time (e.g. 60 minutes) (see Chapter 3).

Note: each of these assessment types requires a practitioner to support, encourage, review, aid understanding and help clarify issues.

What if people can't use books or computers?

Some people like to read and others like to use computers. Yet others prefer not to – or struggle to work in these ways – for example, because of reading problems or lack of access. The Five Areas model is therefore available in a range of ways to encourage accessibility. This includes materials:

- For a range of ages (young people and adults and, shortly, older adults).
- For a range of people (e.g. patients and carers).
- Addressing a range of disorders (e.g. depression, anxiety, panic, postnatal depression, eating disorders, smoking cessation, getting back to work, weight loss, coping with physical symptoms).
- Available in a range of formats (books of different sizes, DVDs, online resources).
- In screen-reader and large print format (for use by people with visual difficulties).
- In a growing range of languages (Chinese Mandarin, simple Chinese text, Bengali, Polish, Dutch, Portuguese, Kurdish – with other languages under way). Many of these are available online under licence. For a list of written resources available in other languages, see Chapter 8.

Licence details for individuals or teams to access the various key Five Areas books online are available at **www.fiveareasonline.com**.

Essential points in the Five Areas assessment

The Five Areas model helps people work out why they feel as they do. The following summarises some of the key elements:

- The Five Areas assessment is a **vicious circle**: All the areas affect each other. This means unhelpful changes can worsen how the patient feels in each area. Importantly it also means that **helpful changes in any of the areas can lead to added benefits in the other areas also**.
- The assessment is the first step needed for change: i.e. the assessment itself can bring about helpful change. Everything in the treatment refers back to the original assessment – which helps inform the short-, medium- and longer-term targets (steps – or in practical terms workbooks or modules) to be worked on.
- Writing down the symptoms/problems matters: it aids engagement and understanding, and facilitates the process of change.
- The assessment is in the patient's own words: this reinforces how the treatment might actually help by changing or improving problem areas. Remember to avoid using jargon and re-summarising what the patient says in technical CBT language.

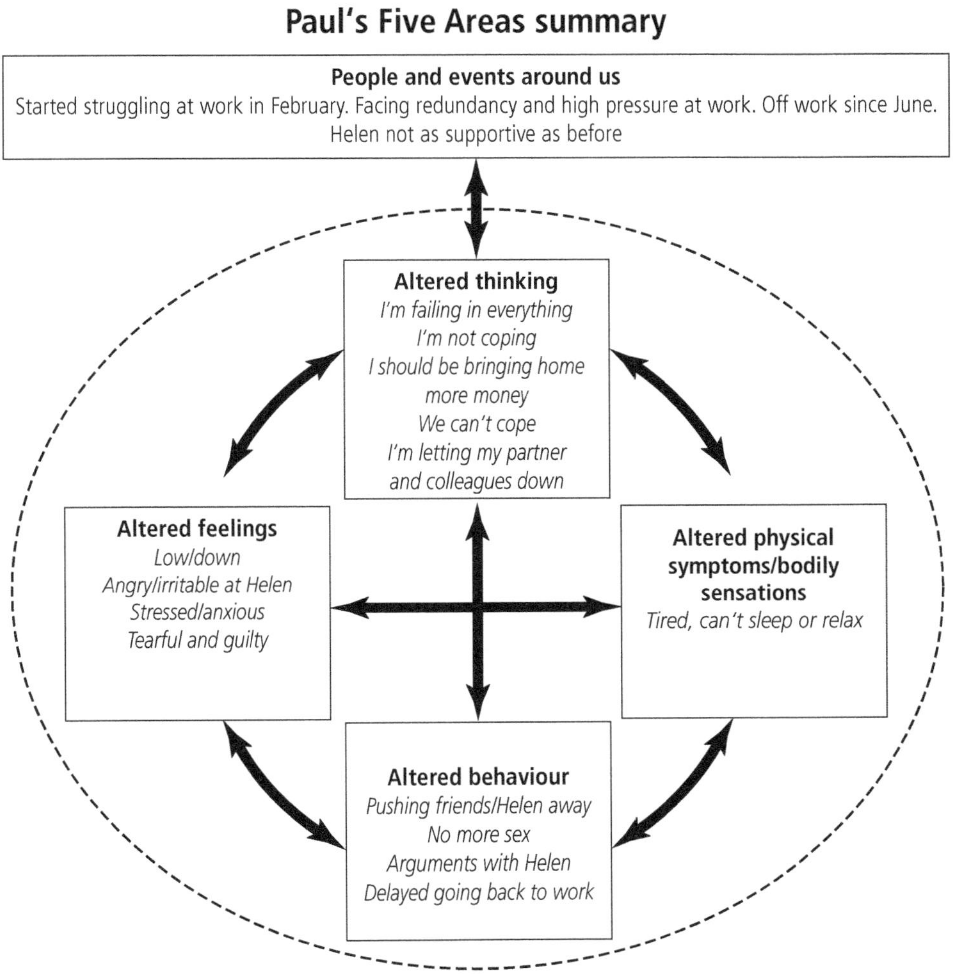

Figure 2.1 The Five Areas summary model used in the Big CBT Books.

It isn't necessary to always identify problems or difficulties in each of the five areas. It is all right leaving a box/area empty. It may be completed at a later date when more information becomes available.

The key is to look for **repeated patterns** of thinking or behaving, and also patterns of emotion (e.g. feeling worse at the start of the day in the diurnal variation often seen during depression), or in particular situations/circumstances (such as when experiencing phobic anxiety) and also patterns of physical symptoms (e.g. more pain when feeling tired or anxious).

The assessment is about identifying potential areas to target for change.

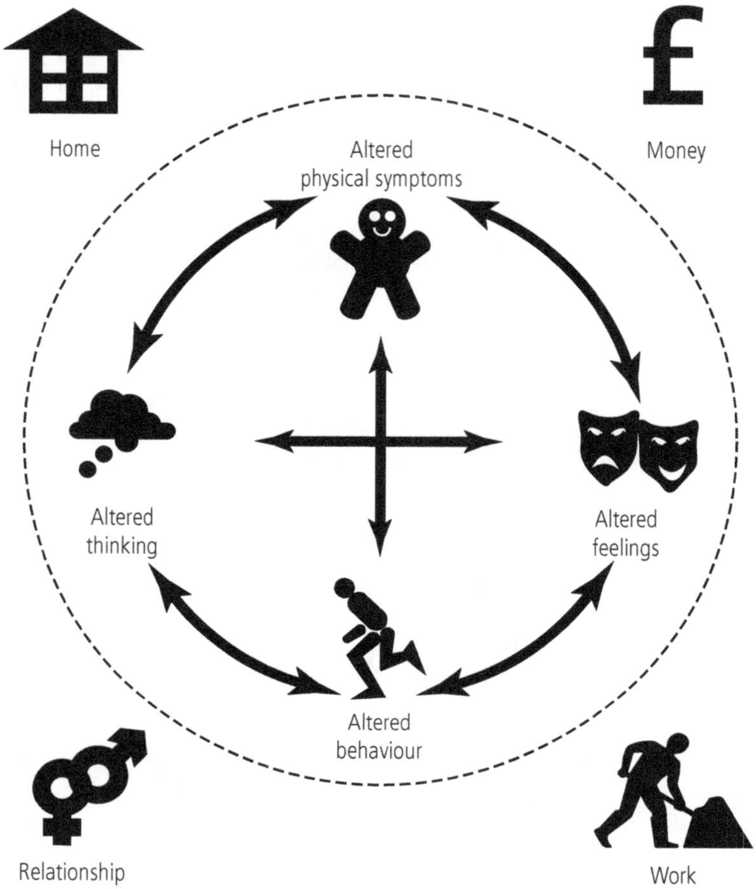

Figure 2.2 The Five Areas icon-style summary model (e.g. as used in the www.llttfi.com package).

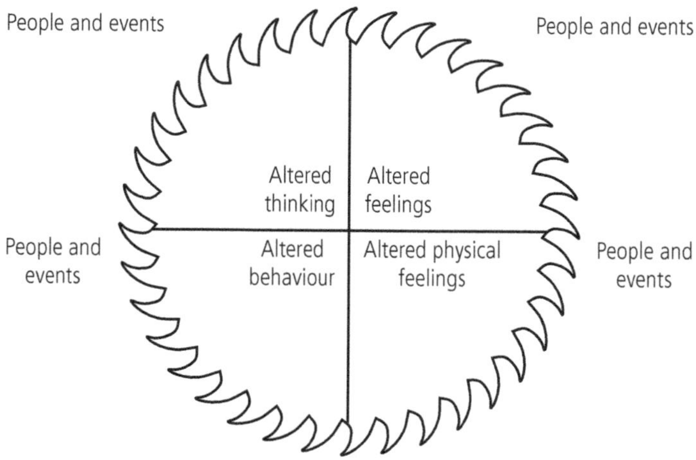

Figure 2.3 The Five Areas vicious circle summary model used in the Little CBT Books.

Key Point

Repeated patterns of thinking, behaviour, emotions or physical symptoms provide the clues as to what needs to change. So, a patient may notice they are prone to certain patterns of thinking (e.g. mind-reading or catastrophising – see below) which occur again and again. Similarly they may note having tummy pain or feeling tense when they are anxious – and noting this again and again whenever they feel anxious. The same principle applies to altered behaviours – where specific repeating patterns such as reduced activity, avoidance or unhelpful behaviours may occur again and again in certain situations or with certain people. Discovering these patterns provides important insight and understanding – but crucially **identifies key targets for change.**

The patient should receive a **written copy** of their own Five Areas assessment. Because it is **their** own assessment, they should be encouraged to modify and amend the content – and keep it constantly up to date. This way the assessment becomes a living and evolving summary of their own problem list that helps target change, update progress and identify next steps to work on.

Communicating the Five Areas model

There are several ways of drawing out and summarising the Five Areas model to engage different people. The different models vary as to how 'visual' and how 'verbal' they are. Three of the models are summarised in Figures 2.1–2.3.

Each of these approaches has a slightly different presentation style, but they all communicate the same basic message: that symptoms can affect each other and a vicious circle can be created – and broken. Blank versions of the first and third structures above are available free of charge from **www.fiveareas.com**.

Patterns of altered thinking

In the traditional CBT model, upsetting thoughts are variously described as *negative automatic thoughts* (automatic because they tend to pop into the patient's mind again and again), or dysfunctional assumptions/schemas/core beliefs. The traditional CBT language also describes a patient as showing cognitive errors or distortions when they are distressed. The problem with such terms is they are complex to learn, difficult to understand, and also run the risk that they are seen as stigmatising and blaming of the patient: 'Great! Not only do I feel really bad – but now they are saying I'm thinking wrongly too!'

In contrast, the Five Areas approach describes such altered thinking as *unhelpful thinking styles*. Seven types of altered thinking occur and are summarised in Table 2.1.

Table 2.1 Unhelpful thinking styles

Unhelpful thinking style	Some typical thoughts
Being your own worst critic/being biased against yourself	• I'm very self-critical • I overlook my strengths • I see myself as not coping • I don't recognise my achievements • I knew that would happen to me!
Putting a negative slant on things (negative mental filter)	• I see things through dark-tinted glasses • I see the glass as being half empty rather than half full • Whatever I've done, it's never enough to give me a sense of achievement • I tend to focus on the bad side of everyday situations
Having a gloomy view of the future (make negative predictions)	• Things will stay bad or just get worse • Things will go wrong • I'm always expecting to fail
Jumping to the worst conclusion (catastrophising)	• I tend to think that the very worst outcome will happen • I often think that I will fail badly
Having a negative view about how others see me (mind-reading)	• I often think that others don't like me or think badly of me without any reason for it
Unfairly taking responsibility for things	• I feel guilty about things even if they aren't really my fault • I think I'm responsible for everyone else
Making extreme statements or rules	• I use the words 'always' and 'never' a lot • If one bad thing happens to me I often say 'just typical' because it seems this always happens • I make myself a lot of 'must', 'should' 'ought' or 'got to' rules

As a practitioner, have you noticed any of these types of thought. Most of us have at least some of them (remember that last appraisal?).

Key Point

Probably most readers of this book will have such thoughts at least some of the time. They are common or normal. Usually, when a person is not feeling depressed or anxious, although they can notice such thoughts, they can quickly put them out of their mind by challenging them – or at least choosing to move on from them. However, during times of anxiety or depression, such thoughts become **more frequent**, and also harder to dismiss. They are also **more believed** – especially at times of high distress. The unhelpful thinking styles matter because they worsen how the patient feels and unhelpfully alter what they do. It is these features that identify a thought that is worth challenging/changing. The various Five Areas thinking workbooks and modules contain tools to help identify such thoughts, and then change them so they become less upsetting.

Patterns of emotions and physical changes

Freud once called dreams the 'royal road to the unconscious'. A similar claim could be made for CBT that 'emotions are the royal road to upsetting thoughts'. One of the most effective interventions in CBT is to identify recurring patterns of thinking and behaviour that keep distress going. For example, when a person suddenly looks upset, anxious, angry, etc., ask 'What's going through your mind right now?' The same approach can be used when a person suddenly notices a strong physical change – for example during panic or pain.

This approach is therefore one of the main tools in the various Five Areas resources to help people identify extreme and upsetting thoughts.

Patterns of altered behaviour

There are three patterns of problematic altered activity – and one helpful pattern. The three vicious circles and one virtuous circle together summarise every response possible when a person is distressed. (This is a big claim – do think it through and see if as a practitioner you can identify any patient responses that cannot be described using the Five Areas circles.) The model can encompass a wide range of so-called maintaining factors that are present in the various disorder-specific CBT models.

Tackling altered behaviour is probably the most effective initial intervention in helping people change. During times of depression and anxiety, phobic anxiety or obsessive-compulsive disorder, it is the avoidance and reduced activity that often has the greatest impact on the patient's life. Because of this, making changes here is an excellent first step for patients to improve their thinking.

Key Point

Helping people with depression increase their activities and get going again is a powerful intervention in overcoming depression. This approach (behavioural activation) can be delivered in a shorter period of time but is as effective as the full CBT approach. See Further reading at the end of the chapter.

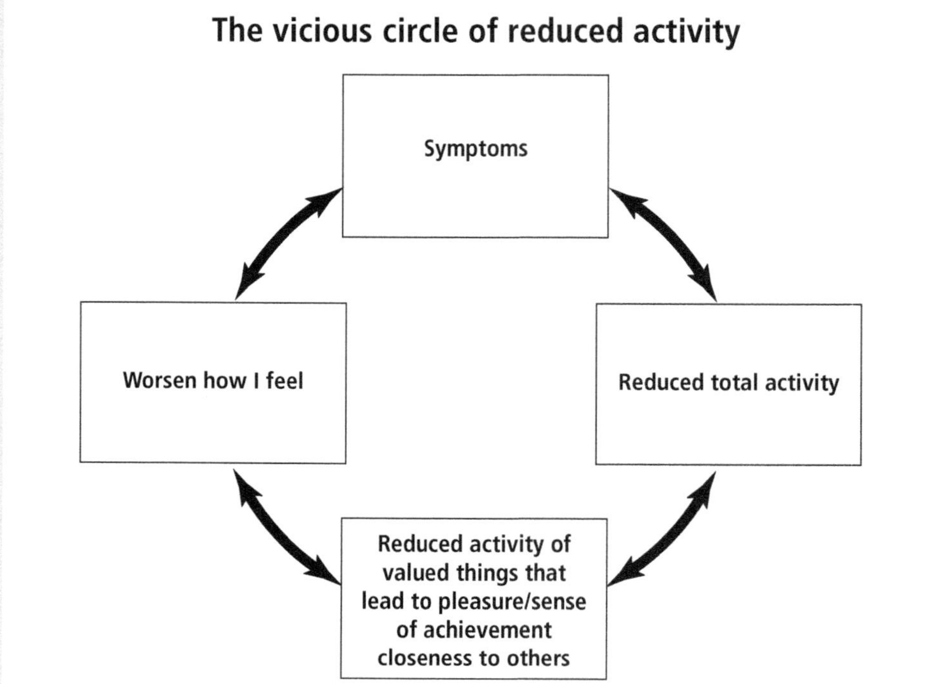

Figure 2.4 The vicious circle of reduced activity.

Key concepts to communicate: 'The less you do, the worse you feel; the worse you feel, the less you do.'

Example of reduced activities: Cutting down on routine things such as ironing and housework, which then build up (distressing), leaving important things undone (e.g. work, paying bills), which cause problems later, reducing the sense of fun/ pleasure in life (e.g. less hobbies) or achievement ('So what, I should be able to do that anyway') and closeness (reduced mixing with friends or going out). The patient either cuts down (early on) or stops doing things completely (later on). All of which (see Fig. 2.4) worsens how the patient feels.

Often at the same time the patient will force themselves to do things they must/ should/ought/got to do (e.g. look after children/go to work). The result is an emptier and emptier and greyer and greyer (sadder) life.

Key point to communicate about making changes: 'Getting going again is important. We need to plan to do something each morning, afternoon and evening.'

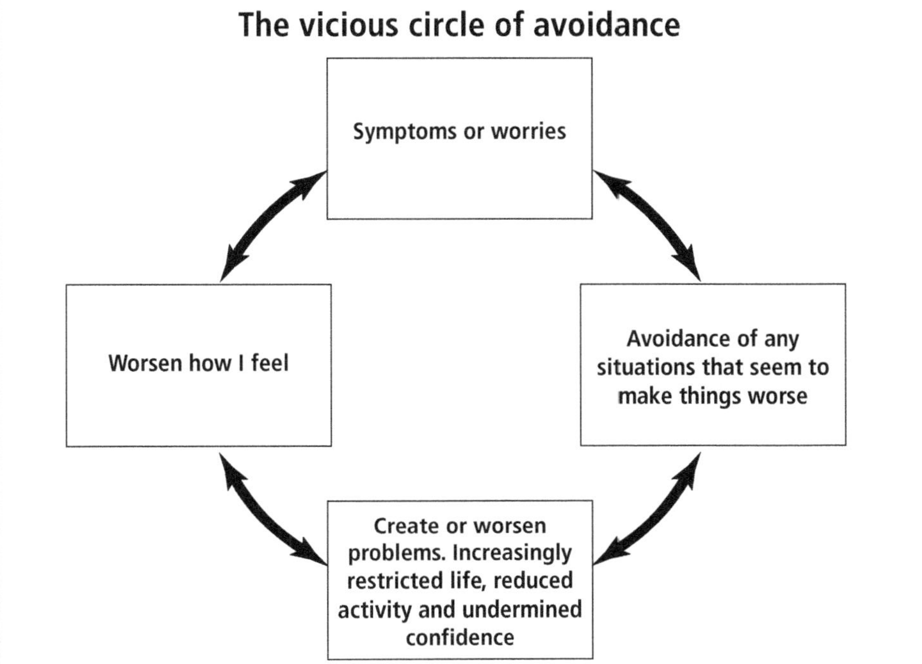

Figure 2.5 The vicious circle of avoidance.

Key concept to communicate: 'It's understandable that when we feel anxious or scared about something, we start to avoid it. The problem is this teaches us that the only way to cope is to avoid something – and slowly, step by step, we lose our confidence even more – and end doing less and less.'

Examples of avoidance: Avoiding visiting 'scary' places such as busy shops or places it is difficult to leave, such as buses and cinemas. There may be avoidance of certain tasks (e.g. driving after an accident), or people/social encounters (social phobia), or certain situations (heights, spiders, enclosed spaces – specific phobias).

Key point to communicate about making changes: 'Confidence is built by planning to face your fears in a step-by-step way. Wouldn't it be great to be able to do these things without worrying about them?'

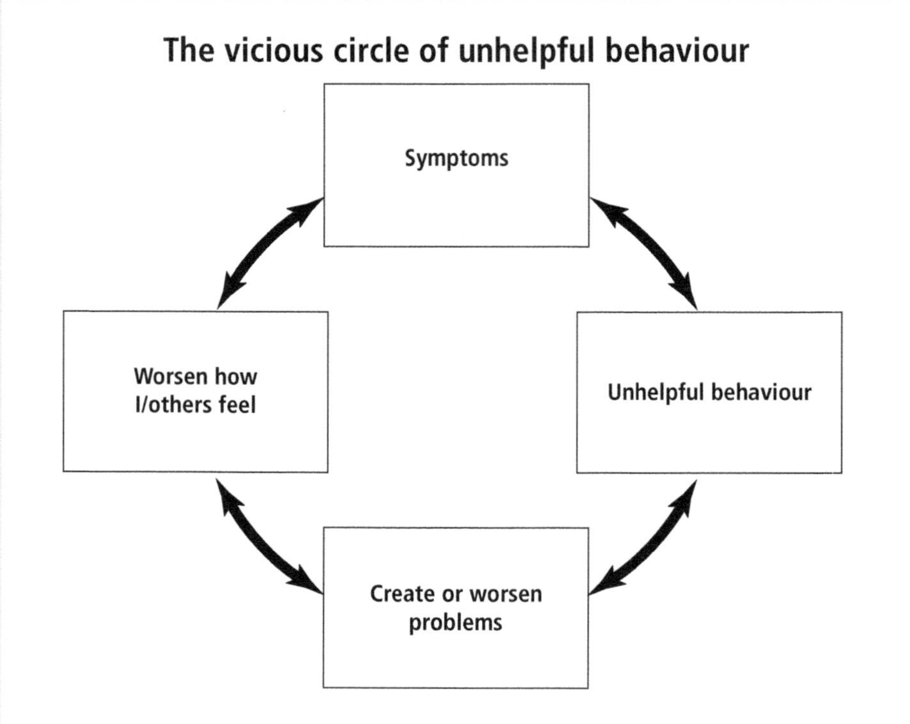

Figure 2.6 The vicious circle of unhelpful behaviour.

Key concepts to communicate: 'When we feel bad it can be tempting to try to block how we feel. People try to do that in all sorts of ways – some helpful and some unhelpful. The problem is that although the unhelpful ways may make us feel better in the short term, in the long term they backfire and make either us – or those around us – feel worse.'

Examples of unhelpful activities: Drinking, smoking or eating to block upsetting feelings. Being rude to others, shouting out or losing their temper unnecessarily may make a patient feel better in the short term but backfire in the longer term. These so-called 'safe' behaviours become part of the problem. The problem is they teach the rule that 'I only managed to cope/survive because I sat down/drank/had taken extra tablets/left', etc. In fact, if they had not done it they would have eventually felt better anyway.

Key point to communicate about making changes: 'We need a clear plan to slowly cut down the unhelpful things you are doing. And at the same time think of some more helpful responses (e.g. tackling upsetting thinking or problem solving).'

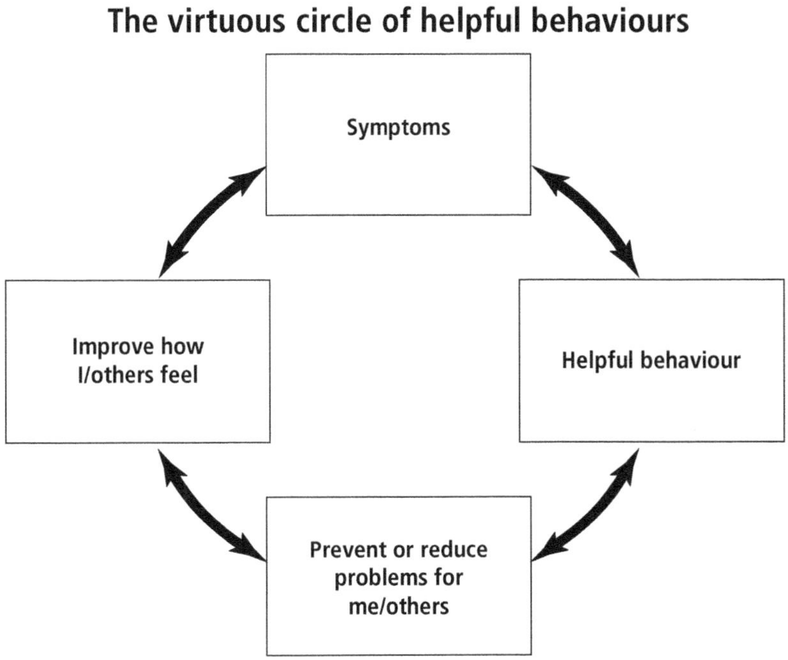

Figure 2.7 The virtuous circle of helpful behaviours.

Key concept to communicate: 'Let's try and work out some things you are doing now – or have done in the past – that will help boost how you feel. We need to get those things working for you in the best way to help you take some more steps forward.'

Example helpful activities: Getting out and about, doing some exercise, eating reasonably healthily, having a haircut, meeting friends, reading CBT self-help resources, seeking support from others whom the patient trusts.

Key point to communicate about making changes: 'It's great there's these things like reading the website that you're doing that is providing useful information. I would like to encourage you to do that. It was interesting looking through your list – I note you have written that you also used to enjoy getting out for walks with your friend. I wondered how you'd feel about trying to start doing that again? If so we could do some planning together about the steps needed to get back to doing that. How does that seem?'

Choosing targets for change

This is expanded on and is a major focus of Chapter 4 (Using the Five Areas assessment to understand why the patient feels as they do). It is important that:

- The choice of area to work on is decided from the joint Five Areas assessment.
- The patient themselves is happy with the choice of target.

Key Point

It is best to choose as the first focus for change something that leads to an **immediate** (or at least fairly rapid, i.e. that week) **benefit** – so that the patient learns something, does something new, or feels even just a bit better. This is needed so that the patient sees a reason to keep working on change. Good first targets include working on sleeping better, taking prescribed medication appropriately and planning to tackle a reduced or avoided activity.

Some more information about the Five Areas approach to changing thinking and behaviour

Each of the various Five Areas resources provides important information about how to change key symptoms. The final part of this chapter focuses on some background information about how and why the Five Areas approach deals with changing altered thoughts and behaviour.

Changing beliefs

In the CBT model, thoughts/beliefs are usually categorised into three different levels:

- Negative automatic thoughts that enter into the mind again and again and cause distress: 'I'll never get the job.' More balanced and accurate thoughts are squeezed out.
- Conditional beliefs such as If … then rules, e.g. '**If** I really open up about who I am, **then** no-one will love me.'
- Schemas/assumptions: That reflect global, all-or-nothing statements such as '**I am** a failure,' '**People are** untrustworthy' or '**The world is** a dangerous place.'

The Five Areas self-help resources aim at working at the level of negative automatic thoughts. They discourage people from using the resources to tackle thoughts that begin with 'I am …', 'People are …' or 'The world is …' (i.e. schemas). Such thoughts require more specialist high intensity CBT interventions (which can be used alongside the self-help approach).

Key Point

Schemas/assumptions can improve significantly by just working at the level of negative automatic thoughts (i.e. extreme and unhelpful thoughts). By helping people catch and respond differently to upsetting thoughts, it is possible to prevent the progression (in CBT terms the 'downward arrow') where one thought quickly cascades down to progressively more and more distressing thoughts and eventually 'hits' a schema. By teaching people the strategies in the Five Areas thinking modules, the patient can be encouraged to respond differently before this happens – thus reducing distress and preventing schema activation.

✓ Practical hints and tips for when working to change extreme and unhelpful thoughts

Not every negative thought is worth challenging. Instead look to work on thoughts that are actually worsening how the patient *feels* – or unhelpfully affecting what they *do*. Encourage the patient to start off with working on thoughts that cause them only mild to moderate distress. This allows them to practise responding to less upsetting thoughts to start with – and build from there.

A range of different interventions are included in the various Five Areas resources. These include mindfulness ('Try not to get caught up in it'), compassionate mind ('What would someone who completely cares for you and is completely on your side say?') as well as the more traditional thought challenge questions ('What advice would you give to a friend who said the same thing?'). Different people will find different aspects of these interventions effective, so it is important to help people practise the different approaches, and eventually settle on a combination that works for them.

The credit card sized thought flashcards (free to download at **www.fiveareas.com**) are a useful pocket resource.

Behavioural experiments as a way of changing beliefs

Although the Five Areas approach doesn't use CBT-related technical language in the resources read by patients, there is a large focus on encouraging people to undermine unhelpful thoughts by acting against them – by using behavioural experiments. In some of the resources the analogy of negative thoughts as a bully is used. By giving in to such thoughts they get built up in the patient's mind and life and become more and more of a problem. Instead the best way to tackle a bully is to face up to it. So – as one book suggests – 'If a thought says don't – then do. If it says can't – then can right back at it.'

By acting against a thought, the Five Areas approach allows the patient to check out exactly what happens when they don't do what it says. This is one of the best ways of undermining negative thoughts. So, if a person is invited to a family event and is tempted to say 'No thanks' because they predict they won't enjoy it, the very best way of finding out if they will or won't enjoy it is to go. Typically (nearly always) things are far better than they thought – especially if they can act against the temptation to arrive late, leave early and sit on the sidelines. Each of these can be aspects of the experiment that is planned ('What might happen if you went up to someone with a big smile and said hello and asked how they were enjoying it'?). The self-help resources encourage such experiments – which can be a powerful way to help people change what they think, feel and do.

Problem solving approaches

Key Point

Research in CBT has shown that when people are depressed or struggling, their ability to problem solve reduces significantly. They are less able to come up with problems – and also tend to discount possible solutions and not follow them up even when they might otherwise have been helpful.

Teaching practical problem solving skills is a key element of the process of change in the Five Areas approach. This is communicated as the **seven-step plan** (Big CBT Books) or **easy four-step plan** (E4SP; Little CBT Books). Both approaches use the same underlying model – but communicate it with different levels of detail.

Comparison of the Big and Little CBT Books problem solving approaches

Big CBT Book approach **Seven steps of problem solving**	**Little CBT Book approach** **Easy four-step plan (E4SP)**
Step 1: Identify and clearly define the problem	Step 1: Break the problem into pieces
Step 2: Think up as many solutions as possible to achieve your first target	Step 2: Brainstorm ways to do the first piece
Step 3: Look at the pros and cons of each possible solution	Step 3: Choose an idea and make a plan to do it
Step 4: Now choose one of the solutions • Will it be useful for changing how you are? • Is it a clear task so that you will know when you've done it? • Is it something that is realistic, practical and achievable?	Step 4: Check the plan and put it into action. Use this checklist: • Is it realistic? • Are you aiming at just one thing? • Is it slow? • Is it easy? • Are you ready to unblock it? Five ticks? Then go for it!
Step 5: Plan the steps needed to carry out your chosen solution. Have you made sure that: • It is clear what you are going to do and when you are going to do it? • Your plan won't be easily blocked or prevented by practical problems? • Your plan will help you to learn useful things even if it doesn't work out perfectly?	
Step 6: Carry out your plan	
Step 7: Review the outcome	

Central to both approaches are:

- A clear and written plan that uses a step-by-step approach.
- Constant review of progress (see the Planner and Review sheets and the Plan, Do, Review Support model in Chapter 5).
- Having back-up plans that predict and aim to overcome potential problems and blocks.
- Taking a non-blaming and problem solving approach if difficulties arise.
- When using the self-help books, ensure the patient has the accompanying worksheet handouts of the E4SP and a blank seven-steps worksheet to help practise the approach again and again (downloadable from **www.fiveareas.com** and **www.fiveareasonline.com**.

Changing behaviour

The seven-step problem solving plan (Big CBT Books) and the E4SP (Little CBT Books) can be used to tackle any problem as well as to help bring about changes in behaviour:

✔ Practical hints and tips for tackling reduced activity

Encourage the patient to use the seven-step plan (described on page 26) to plan:

1. Things that give a sense of pleasure, achievement or closeness.
2. The routine things that will build up otherwise and make the patient feel worse (e.g. ironing, weeding).
3. Essential things that otherwise upset the patient or make them feel worse (e.g. paying bills where possible – even in part – to avoid falling into arrears and facing the added stresses this will bring).

Key problem to overcome in planning change

When patients try to go too fast – by planning to take steps that are too ambitious so planned changes that seem too much/scary/hard – remind them: 'You're not trying to run a marathon are you?'

✔ Practical hints and tips for tackling aviodance: ideas to guide the content of change

Use the seven-step plan (or E4SP) described on page 26. 'We need to plan to face the fears slowly – so that you get really good at doing things before moving on. Each step needs to move forward – and push you – but not so much to make you feel it's too fast or too scary and just want to give up.'

Key problem to overcome in planning change

Avoidance can be quite subtle. For example the patient goes out with a mobile not just because they might get a call – but instead 'just in case something happens'. Similarly, the patient joins the shortest queue at the shops because it allows them to escape quickly rather than because it is the sensible thing to do.

✓ Practical hints and tips for tackling unhelpful behaviours: ideas to guide the content of change

Encourage the patient to use the seven steps of problem solving or the E4SP to cut down just one unhelpful behaviour.

Key problem to overcome in planning change

Sometimes people think that drinking, shouting, etc. is part of the solution. This is because they haven't worked out that such behaviours actually add to the problem. A helpful strategy is to ask the following questions to help people work out for themselves again and again the costs/downsides of some of these behaviours:

- 'What impact did that immediately have on you physically, psychologically (in your thinking and emotions) and on what you did?'
- 'How about later? What was the impact then?'
- 'What about how it affected others/what others did/said/how they reacted?'

Often people focus on the short-term benefits but completely overlook the longer-term costs. By going through times when the problematic behaviour (e.g. drinking too much) may have occurred again and again – and slowing down the discussion to tease out the negatives, people can slowly get to understand the unhelpful impact of such patterns of behaviour.

Resources for change

This section provides an overview of the book-based resources that address the topics covered in this chapter. These are expanded on in Chapter 8. DVD and web-based versions are also available and are described in more detail in Chapter 9.

Five Areas assessment

- Little CBT Books: *Why do I feel so bad?*; *How to use the Little CBT Books – a practitioner's guide*.
- Big CBT Books: e.g. *Understanding why you feel as you do*.

Problem solving

- Little CBT Books: *How to fix almost everything*.
- Big CBT Books: *Practical problem solving*.

Altered thinking

- Little CBT Books: *Why does everything always go wrong?*
- Big CBT Books: *Noticing and changing extreme and unhelpful thinking*.

Altered behaviour

- Little CBT Books: *The things you do that mess you up; I can't be bothered doing anything*.
- Big CBT Books: *Doing things that boost how you feel; Using exercise to boost how you feel; Helpful things you can do; Unhelpful things you do; Overcoming anxiety and avoidance*.

Completing a Five Areas assessment without changing everything you do as a practitioner

Some practitioners focus their entire discussion on the completion of a Five Areas assessment, and this provides the main structure to their assessment. Such an approach is outlined in Chapters 3 and 4. However, it is also possible to complete a Five Areas assessment as an additional add-on to the usual assessment process a practitioner would undertake, whatever their background.

So, for example, if the practitioner is a nurse, a doctor, a psychologist, an occupational therapist, a teacher or a social worker – or from a range of varied health or social care workers, they will already be highly skilled in doing a structured assessment. This probably covers the same five areas as in the Five Areas model and more, but the practitioner will most likely structure the summary of the assessment differently depending on their training. This is because most assessments enquire about how people feel, what they are concerned about, what is going on in their life, how it is affecting them emotionally and physically and how they live their life and cope. Different professional groups may emphasise one or more areas, but all five areas tend to be covered at least to some extent at some stage.

Key Point

It is possible to complete an assessment/screen/meeting with a patient in the usual way, but by watching out for the symptoms/problems in each of the five areas. By jotting them down on a blank Five Areas sheet as the interview proceeds, the practitioner can create a Five Areas assessment to discuss and work on together.

Common questions about using the Five Areas assessment

What if the patient becomes distressed when they see their assessment?

Most people find it helpful and empowering to see their symptoms written down on paper or on a computer screen. For the first time they begin to see how things relate to each other and that change is possible. Sometimes, however, when the patient sees their various symptoms written down, they suddenly realise quite how much the low mood etc. is affecting them and feel more distressed as a result. This is why it is important that appropriate support is offered by a practitioner. Key things that could be said in this circumstance are:

- 'These symptoms/problems were already there **before** the assessment – they are not new. At least now you know about them and can start to do something to change things.'
- 'I'm here to work with you – and together we can get a plan that helps change things around.'
- 'If it all seems too much, why don't we focus on just one single area to start with? Small steady steps can really help and it's surprising how working on just one thing can quite quickly lead to benefits in other areas too.'

What about the past?

The Five Areas model aims to provide a summary of the current problems facing the patient. Some patients will have experienced traumatic or other upsetting events in the past that continue to affect them even now. They may lead to upsetting memories, thoughts or repeated patterns of behaviour (e.g. constantly seeking out violent partners because of previous childhood experiences of abuse). These would be summarised on their Five Areas model and are examples of how the past affects the present. This emphasises the importance of watching for recurrent patterns in how the patient thinks, feels and responds, all of which act to make them feel worse.

Using the Five Areas assessment in busy teams and for CPA

Practitioners often work as part of teams where large parts of team meetings focus on the practitioners feeding back new patient assessments. This can be appropriate; however, the process can be given a fresh impetus and a real focus by using the Five Areas model as a format for feedback. This can be done in several ways:

- Handing round a photocopy of the Five Areas assessment of a new patient, and talking for a maximum of five minutes about the key symptoms, development and other relevant information.
- The same information can be provided as a presentation using a laptop projected on to a wall, similar to the use of acetate and overhead projectors in past years when summarising a clinical case (remember those?).
- This approach provides an invaluable but simple summary that can accompany letters to the general practitioner (GP) and other referrers.
- In CPA (care programme approach) meetings, where there are multiple issues/problems, the Five Areas assessment can helpfully summarise who or which agency is working on each specific problem area.
- At times of staff changeover (e.g. when new staff members join a team, or old staff move on) the Five Areas assessment provides a useful handover note.

The Five Areas assessment also works well as a quick aide memoire of current symptoms and can be used as a reminder when seeing patients for intermittent (e.g. six monthly or annual) reviews. At that frequency of contact one can easily forget or overlook important problem areas, and a summary diagram at the front of the clinical case record can help focus the review meeting and allow a rapid current update and review.

Advanced skills

When first starting out using the Five Areas approach it can sometimes feel enough just asking the questions to identify current problems and symptoms. However, there are substantial benefits of also working with the patient to identify current or past personal strength areas/resources. This can involve asking questions such as: 'What would you have done in the past to deal with this sort of problem?' or 'If you weren't feeling like this, what would you want to do here to tackle this situation?'

A helpful approach is to use the Five Areas assessment to also examine times when the patient feels better so as to identify helpful patterns of responding that can be built on.

Task

- Go through the Five Areas assessment as usual to identify the patient's problematic thoughts and behaviours, for example by focusing on understanding specific times when they have felt worse, lower, sadder, angrier, more in pain/tired or more anxious/scared.
- Remember to also go through some examples of when they feel better, happier, smiling, calmer, less in pain/more energetic and more relaxed. Again look for helpful patterns that can be built on or hidden avoidance – where the patient feels better because they are overtly or covertly (mentally) avoiding doing something that seems scary.
- A further area sometimes overlooked or relatively ignored in assessment is understanding and helping people respond to external problems and relationships. Most people feel like they do for a reason. Tackling some of these reasons directly or sign-posting people to somewhere they can obtain that help is an important part of recovery.

The Five Areas approach in high intensity CBT

As mentioned earlier in this chapter, the Five Areas language and style of communicating the CBT model can be used in low intensity (limited practitioner contact) and high intensity (longer and more sessions) settings.

Key Point

The Five Areas assessment and language can be decoupled from the idea of using the various Five Areas self-help resources. In other words, the practitioner can use the Five Areas assessment approach and language, and communicate the model wholly verbally – or with just a few key Five Areas handouts (such as the vicious circle sheets and unhelpful thinking styles sheets) rather than using the wider range of Five Areas self-help resources. The same is true for a person struggling to use, or who doesn't want to use, self-help resources. The key to any working is engaging and working with the patients in the way they need and want to work. However, if choosing to work in this way, we recommend that practitioners have a wider working knowledge of the CBT model so that the interventions continue to be informed by the evidence-based CBT approach.

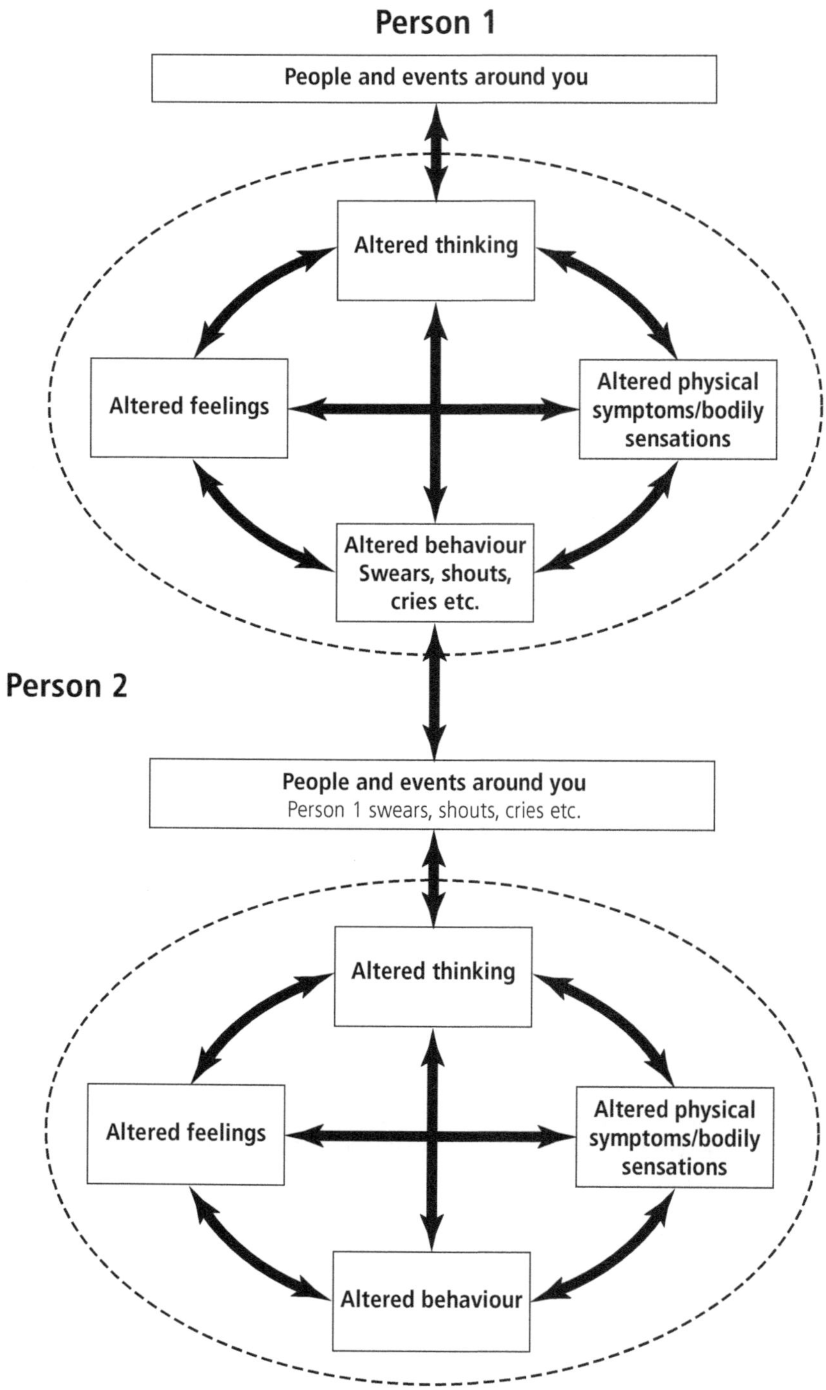

Figure 2.8 Using the Five Areas model in systemic CBT.

Think about how a person responds using the Five Areas assessment. One area is their behaviour. Now imagine a second person who is in the same room as that first person when they carry out that behaviour. For example person 1 shouts or cries or swears. For person 2, that behaviour is the situation, people or events around them. Two interlocking vicious circles can therefore be set up. This approach allows systemic factors to be conceptualised within a Five Areas model, which can be helpful in a range of settings such as working with young people and for understanding carer and staff responses to upsetting patients (such as in dementia wards and personality difficulties wards).

There are various Five Areas resources aimed at carers including chapters in books (carer workbooks in *Overcoming depression and low mood,* and *Overcoming teenage low mood and depression*) and websites (e.g. **www.overcominganorexiaonline.com**).

Online training resources

There are several Five Areas websites offering training, resources and other useful information for practitioners:

- Visit **www.fiveareas.com** for access to the whole range of Five Areas resources including free downloads. Books and translations are available here.
- **www.fiveareastraining.com** has a range of online modules addressing the Five Areas course.
- **www.livinglifetothefull.com** (short-cut **www.llttf.com**) has all the key modules practitioners need to get going and to use the popular Living Life to the Full course. It also has practitioner training resources for the Plan, Do, Review model and a Quick Start guide to using the course.

Key practice points

- The Five Areas approach provides a summary of problems described in terms of a vicious circle.
- Making changes in any area can be beneficial.
- Choosing targets that have an early positive impact (such as overcoming sleep problems, taking medication regularly or focusing on behavioural activation) are all good first steps.
- Crucially the patient themselves needs to choose the first step for change.
- The Five Areas model is not a new model of CBT. Instead it aims to communicate key CBT principles around understanding, changing thinking and behaviour in a simple and straightforward way.

Next steps

- Complete the free online practitioner training modules at **www.livinglifetothefull.com** or **www.llttf.com**
- Then see the additional training modules for practitioners at **www.fiveareastraining.com**.

Further reading

Cuijpers P, van Straten A, Warmerdam L. (2007) Behavioral activation treatments of depression: A meta-analysis. *Clinical Psychology Review* **27**: 318–26.

Dimidjian S, Hollon SD, Dobson KS, Schmaling KB *et al.* (2006) Randomized trial of behavioral activation, cognitive therapy, and antidepressant medication in the acute treatment of adults with major depression. *Journal of Consulting and Clinical Psychology* **74**: 658–70.

Garland A, Fox R, Williams CJ. (2002) Overcoming reduced activity and avoidance: a five areas approach. *Advances in Psychiatric Treatment* **8**: 6, 453–62.

Williams C, Garland A. (2002) Identifying and challenging unhelpful thinking. *Advances in Psychiatric Treatment* **8**: 377–86.

Williams CJ, Garland A. (2002) A cognitive behavioural therapy assessment model for use in everyday clinical practice. *Advances in Psychiatric Treatment* **8**: 172–9.

Wright B, Williams C, Garland A. (2002) Using the five areas cognitive-behavioural therapy model with psychiatric patients. *Advances in Psychiatric Treatment* **8**: 307–15.

PART 2

Using the Five Areas approach

Chapter 3

Completing a collaborative Five Areas assessment

What you will learn

In this first of two chapters addressing clinical assessment you will learn about:

- The ways in which you can complete a collaborative Five Areas assessment.
- Alternative ways of carrying out assessments in 10, 30 and 60 minutes.
- Using the Five Areas assessment to create a summary of symptoms/problems over the past two weeks.
- How the concept of diagnosis overlaps with a Five Areas assessment.
- How the Five Areas model can help identify key symptoms in a range of common mental and physical health disorders.

Chapter 4 will focus on how to complete a Five Areas assessment to help understand specific times when the patient has felt worse.

Carrying out assessments

Think about the last time you underwent some form of healthcare assessment. How did you feel at that time? For most people, an assessment can be an uncomfortable process to go through, and anxiety levels can rise.

Q Think back in your own life to consultations you have had with a healthcare worker. Have any such contacts been either helpful and supportive, or unsupportive or otherwise unhelpful in some way? What made the difference between the two?

This raises the question: What makes a good assessment? Were you clear about why you were asked the questions that were put to you in your own assessment? Or even why you were there in the first place and how that practitioner might have been able to help you? Did they explain what the assessment was for and how the information that you gave to them would be used?

In nearly every service, whether in the National Health Service (NHS), or the voluntary or private sector, a patient usually undergoes some form of initial assessment before treatment begins. As a worker undertaking frequent assessments, sometimes several in a day, it can be easy to forget exactly how difficult this can be for each individual concerned. Assessment can become simply a service-driven process bound by protocols and tradition. The same questions are often asked of every patient, sometimes with limited explanation and led by the clinician. At the same time, the questions asked often address very personal situations and emotions and the patient is asked to confide all of this to a relative stranger whom they may have met only moments before for the first time (or indeed never met if the initial assessment is conducted over the telephone).

The patient's view of assessment

From the perspective of the patient attending the assessment, they may have answered similar questions many times before, asked by many different people. Therefore it can be frustrating for them that the information is being requested again. All of this can also be compounded by their current emotional state and associated symptoms. They may also have symptoms of pain, or may struggle to concentrate during the assessment due to anxiety or as a symptom of low mood.

Lack of motivation and energy may cause significant problems of engagement. It can be difficult for a patient to engage in an assessment fully if they are experiencing significant negative thinking and are feeling hopeless and helpless about the future and their current situation. This may precipitate negative thoughts about the appointment and the practitioner, and may affect any potential future benefits of engaging with the treatment. These thoughts therefore need to be actively addressed during the first appointment and reinforce the need for the patient to feel understood, and to choose a target to work on that is agreed as being relevant by themselves.

The practitioner's perspective of the assessment

When learning new skills, practitioners may also be anxious about completing and undertaking clinical assessments. There can be a lot of information that needs to be gathered, and practitioners have the task of not only empathically listening to what is being said but also trying to make sense of it. They also need to, all at the same time, link all the gathered information together and think about how they can help the patient, and the resources they may offer the patient to do this. This process of assessment and integration of what is discovered is a complex skill, and like any skill it needs practice.

During the early stages of training, clinicians understandably find it difficult to focus on what question to ask next, while also taking notes, being empathic and trying to listen attentively. At this stage in development of assessment skills, use of a crib sheet or assessment sheet can help with this process and build confidence.

Key Point

As with learning to drive, it can be helpful to practise doing assessments using a clear structure that is repeated again and again. In this way, the practitioner's focus will eventually move away from getting the structure right to instead focus on what is being said and how it is communicated.

Completing a Five Areas assessment in 10, 30 and 60 minutes

Practitioners reading this book will be working in a range of different settings and will have a variety of different session lengths available for conducting their assessments and gathering information. This section of the chapter therefore focuses on completing an assessment in 10, 30 and 60 minutes.

Assessments in 10 minutes

Ten-minute assessments are done in situations where there are large numbers of patients, such as advice/drop-in clinics or routine appointments in general practice.

Here the assessment can be helpfully structured using a single Five Areas assessment worksheet. Free Five Areas summary worksheets (see Chapter 1) are available from **www.fiveareas.com**. These provide a useful structure to quickly assess how the patient has been feeling recently.

The Five Areas assessment can focus on one of two things:

- A recent time when the patient has felt worse. This helps identify typical patterns of thinking and behaviour – and to start establishing if these are problem patterns that are recurring. This is the focus of Chapter 4.
- How the patient has felt in general over the past two weeks. This helps the practitioners come up with an overall **diagnosis/problem** statement of the problems being faced.

When time is this short, aim to identify several key problem areas – and begin to introduce how thoughts, feelings, physical symptoms and behaviour all tie together. In 10 minutes sometimes only part of the Five Areas assessment diagram may be completed – so it may be revisited over several short contacts – thereby allowing more detail to be added. It can be thought of as *working formulation* that can be added to subsequently, and serves as a reminder to the practitioner to ask more about a certain area the next time they see the patient.

If the practitioner is not sure if something is a problem for the patient, or there isn't time to enquire in detail, they can put a question mark in the box as a memory jogger for themselves or for the patient to take away and think more about and add to their diagram before the next meeting. See Figure 3.1 for an example.

Five Areas assessment information gathered in 10 minutes

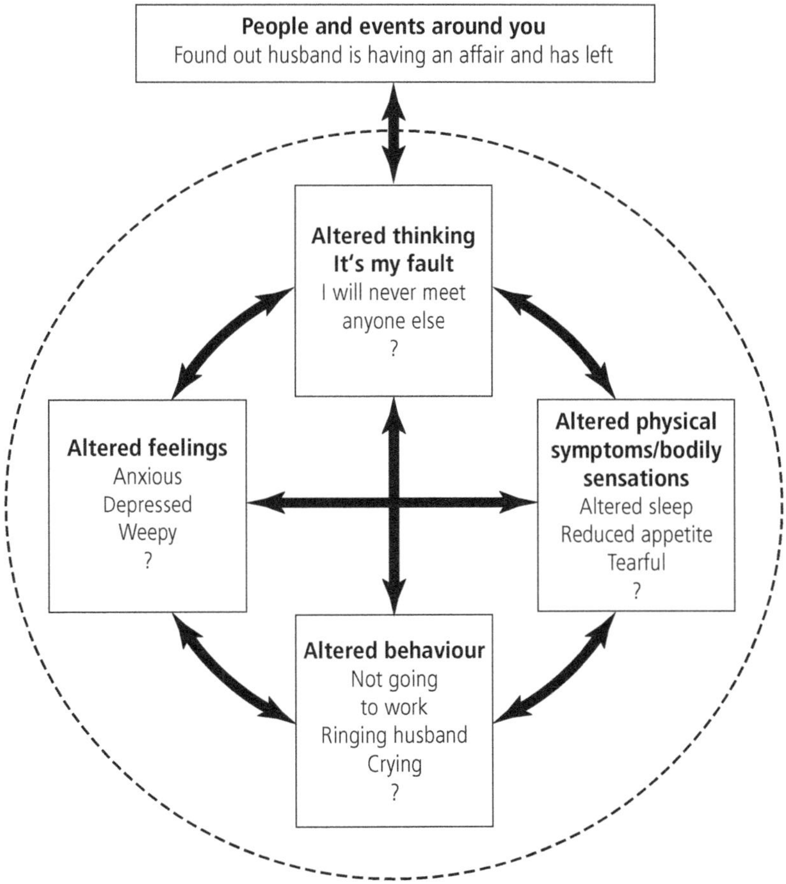

Figure 3.1 Five Areas assessment information gathered in 10 minutes.

Remember, although 10 minutes provides only limited time, it is still important to give the patient the chance to look at the diagram and to talk through one or two key elements of the model, and to ideally take home a copy of their own written assessment summary sheet.

Book- or online-based self-assessment

Practitioners often believe that doing an assessment always means sitting down and completing it together. However, most patients are more than able to work out themselves how they are feeling – and the Five Areas resources provide them with a useful structure to do this. The advantage of the Five Areas guided cognitive behavioural therapy (CBT) resources is that each resource approach also includes a self-assessment component that the patient can complete on their own at home. Table 3.1 lists some of the self-assessment modules in a range of the Five Areas books.

Table 3.1 Five Areas self-assessment book resources (resources not in italics are out of print)

Five Areas guided CBT self-help resource	Module/workbook name
Overcoming anxiety, stress and panic, 2nd edition	*Understanding worry and stress*
	Understanding panic and phobias
Overcoming depression and low mood, 3rd edition	*Understanding why you feel as you do*
Overcoming postnatal depression	*Understanding why you feel as you do*
Overcoming teenage low mood and depression	*Understanding why I feel as I do*
Little CBT Books series:	
Why do I feel so bad?	
I'm not supposed to feel like this	
What anxiety and depression are and how they affect us	
Overcoming anxiety, 1st edition	Workbook 1a: Understanding how anxiety is affecting me
	Workbook 1b: Understanding worry and generalised anxiety
	Workbook 1c: Understanding panic and phobias
	Workbook 1d: Understanding obsessive compulsive symptoms
	Workbook 1e: Understanding how we respond to physical health problems
Overcoming depression and low mood, 2nd edition	*Understanding why I feel as I do*

Each of the self-assessment books in Table 3.1 has linked black and white or full colour worksheets in which the patient can summarise their problems using a Five Areas assessment. These worksheets can be downloaded free of charge from **www.fiveareas.com**.

Key Point

The workbooks in the Five Areas books help people to do a self-assessment/ formulation. The patient can then show their Five Areas summary to the practitioner at the next appointment. In online computerised CBT (cCBT) courses such as **www.llttfi.com** the patient can print out their own personalised Five Areas assessment, and this assessment helps define what subsequent module components are worked on so that the package addresses their own specific symptoms.

The patient presents with a clear and focused request for treatment

The patient may present with a clearly identified problem, e.g. 'I'm not sleeping well'. In this case the brief assessment is focused on identifying whether just to go straight to handing out the focused workbook on sleep problems, or whether there may be other important problems that need to be addressed. Is the sleep problem part of depression, a crisis situation, a symptom of a physical disorder (such as night-time asthma) or some other problem such as alcohol dependence? In the limited time available it is therefore important the practitioner asks appropriate, brief screening questions aimed at identifying other common mental and physical health problems that may account for the presenting symptom, or arrange a longer time to allow a fuller assessment by an appropriate practitioner.

Key Point

A 10-minute assessment should focus on how symptoms are affecting the patient right now/recently and aim to identify a target for change and/or establish a likely diagnosis.

Assessment in 30 minutes

In 30 minutes you have a lot more time to explore the symptoms and their impact.

Key Point

Thirty-minute assessments focus on how symptoms are affecting the patient right now, and they can also explore the development of symptoms and factors that help or worsen how the patient feels. The assessment will still cover the same areas as in the 10-minute assessment; however, there is much more time to help the patient understand the model, and how different symptoms relate as part of a vicious circle. The longer session allows more time for discussion, checking understanding and making collaborative decisions about choosing targets and next steps.

A blank Five Areas assessment question sheet can again help structure the assessment.

Assessment in 60 minutes

Here, there is far more time and the work clinically is likely to be in a specialist counselling or psychotherapy setting (either high or low intensity setting).

Key Point

In 60-minute assessments there is time for a more detailed discussion of current and past problems, the development of the current problems and factors influencing how the patient feels. Usually this would lead to a full CBT formulation.

In a typical longer assessment, the practitioner can ask about all sorts of details of how problems have developed (e.g. as a timeline – see the workbook *Understanding why you feel as you do* in *Overcoming depression and low mood*). In addition, key points from the patient's life history are asked about and help make sense of the rules they have learned about how they see and judge themselves, others and the world around them, and of the responses and problem solving strategies (helpful or unhelpful) they have learned in the past and continue to use today.

Overview of realistic goals of what can be achieved in 10, 30 and 60 minute assessments

	Just 10 minutes	30 minutes	60 minutes
Establishing relationship	+	++	++
Effective communications skills (checking understanding etc.)	+	++	+++
Five Areas assessment	(+) Book/cCBT based or very short	++	+++
Detailed description of how the five areas affect each other	+	++	+++
Understand current problems	+	++	+++
Recent problems (past two weeks)	+	++	+++
Understand problems from the past (childhood)	–	–/+	+++
Development of problems/timeline/factors affecting symptoms	Via books	+	++
Check for other mental/physical health problems	+	+	+
Check for risk	+ E.g. use of standard risk times on questionnaire	+	+

Purpose of an assessment

Assessment is the opportunity for the patient to begin to understand why they currently feel as they do. It is also the first step of treatment and identifies targets for change. It crucially helps build the therapeutic relationship – one of the most important factors that affect outcome.

Assessment is firstly about the individual and is their pivotal first step in treatment. It should foster hope that change is possible – and give a sense of control in the process to the patient themselves. The patient is the expert when it comes to their own experiences; no one has experienced the difficulties they face in their own unique way. In an assessment process the patient is choosing to open up and share these experiences, with the hope that the assessor might be able to offer help and support, and to make them feel better.

Assessment is an educative process that enables the patient to see what it is that they are currently doing that is helpful, as well as identifying things that are not so helpful and are making them distressed. Often patients come with expectations that practitioners will 'do something' or offer a cure. Adopting a stance where practitioners see their role as teachers and motivators in helping the patient work on their own change is central to the Five Areas approach. To a large extent change is down to the individual themselves and is an active process on their part. Practitioners should offer guidance, support and motivation to use a range of evidence-based techniques that the patient is likely to benefit from, and offer hope that (realistic) change is possible and that it is within their control.

Relationships – the role of 'common factors'

'Common factors' are factors that are common across a range of evidence-based approaches and have a beneficial effect on outcome. These include, for example, verbal and non-verbal communication skills such as:

- Warmth, empathy and genuineness.
- Displaying understanding and interest in the patient with frequent summaries and paraphrasing, making eye contact and using nods and gestures to display the practitioner's interest if in a face-to-face session. The equivalent in telephone support would be 'hmm' and 'yes' statements coupled with frequent short summaries, for example: 'Okay, so you are finding it difficult at the moment and have told me your mood is really down, and this has affected your energy levels and is causing problems with your sleep and at work – have I got that right?' An example of using paraphrasing to show you are listening is: 'Earlier you told me that you had stopped going to see your friend Julie. Is there anything else you have stopped doing since you have felt this way?'

Diagnosis and the Five Areas approach

The Five Areas assessment helps the patient identify the impact of low mood, depression, physical problems or life crises etc. on the five key aspects of their life. It presents a detailed summary of how the symptoms are affecting the patient. This gives information about the patient and their difficulties that is far more functionally useful than a short diagnostic label/summary or a written problem statement.

However, the concept of diagnosis can be helpful in other ways. For example, it allows professionals to communicate quickly, and is widely used in research settings. The CBT approach therefore has tended to see diagnoses as being compatible and as sitting alongside more detailed case summaries/case formulations such as the Five Areas assessment. Consequently, the aim of the assessment is to create a shared understanding of the presenting problem, to make psychological sense of this, and to identify targets for change in the respective areas. Crucially, it is created equally for use by the patient as well as for the practitioner.

For example, Table 3.2 summarises the key differences between generalised anxiety and other anxiety disorders.

Table 3.2 Disorder specific changes in different mental health presentations.

	Thinking	Feelings	Physical symptoms	Behaviour
Generalised anxiety disorder	Worrying	On edge Stressed Irritable Not enjoying things/low	Tiredness, mild somatic symptoms, sleeplessness	Fidgety, avoid/put things off, mild checking Reassurance seeking + Blocking feelings with drink/smoking/seeking excessive reassurance from others
Panic attacks/ phobic fear	Believing that something catastrophic is happening right now, e.g. going to collapse, suffocate, die	Panicky Terrified	Hyperventilation, rapid heart, sweaty, clammy, shaky, sick, feeling dizzy/ depersonalised, dry mouth	Leave suddenly and avoid in future Reassurance seeking ++ Safety behaviours to reduce anxiety or fear of worse thing happening, e.g. sitting down when feeling dizzy to avoid collapse, carrying water to avoid dry mouth Block feelings with drink/ smoking
Depression	Negative view of self, situation and the future	Down/low Anxious No enjoyment (anhedonia)	Somatic/endogenous/ biological symptoms of depression, e.g. weight loss, loss of appetite, low energy, agitation, restlessness, poor sleep, loss of sex drive, constipation, poor or increased appetite and weight, reduced activity or mild over-activity	Unhelpful behaviours to block mood, e.g. smoking/ drinking Reduced activity
Obsessive compulsive symptoms	Predicting something terrible will happen Feeling personally responsible for preventing this occurring	Anxious Scared/panicky Low Irritable Guilty	Anxiety symptoms On edge, rapid heart, tense, weary, etc.	Anxious preoccupation Safety behaviours Reversing behaviours Cleaning/checking/ counting rituals Mental rituals, e.g. prayers, doing things a set number of times.

In understanding the CBT model, it is helpful to remember that CBT provides *disorder-specific models* for understanding symptoms. This means that particular disorders present in different ways in each of the Five Areas. Different clinical diagnoses therefore require different interventions in line with this. So the factor that makes depression and not generalised anxiety disorder (GAD) is that each has different symptom patterns. It also explains why some symptoms overlap across diagnoses (and hence why the concept of diagnosis is fundamentally flawed). So, for example, up to 70 per cent of people with depressive disorder also have significant anxiety symptoms. This is where the idea of themes and typical behaviour changes/patterns (vicious circles) can be useful.

Key symptoms in different mental health disorders

Certain disorders have general 'themes' and manifest as typical vicious circles of altered behaviour.

Generalised anxiety disorder

In GAD, there is low-level anxiety that may be present a lot of the time (generalised). Physical symptoms include headaches, pains, tiredness and poor sleep. Often the person is facing a range of external issues, problems or hassles related to, for example, money, job, relationships, or worries about other external challenges such as exams.

People with GAD have significant worry about more than one area of their life and have an intolerance of uncertainty, unpredictability and situations in which they feel a lack of control and uncertainty. They not only may have positive beliefs about the worrying being helpful ('Worrying helps me keep control', 'If I didn't worry then I would fall apart') but also may have negative beliefs about the fact they worry so much and what this means to them ('I am going mad', 'I am going crazy', 'If I don't stop worrying then I will lose my mind').

Altered behaviours include avoidance leading to a restricted life and reduced confidence. People with GAD may have poor problem solving skills, and may try to avoid thinking about anxiety provoking situations, or avoid entering situations which they feel are uncertain or unpredictable or that they cannot control, or struggle with a worsening of their anxiety levels when they do attempt these things – for example, moving home, going away to university, starting a new relationship.

Indulgence in unhelpful behaviours to try to block the anxiety is common, including drinking, smoking and eating, and irritability at self and others.

Figure 3.2 illustrates how GAD affects the five areas of life.

Depression and low mood

A theme in depression is that of actual or perceived losses. An *actual loss* may be present, such as a bereavement or loss of a job. A *perceived loss* might be a loss of status or role, for example a parent whose child has left home to go to university and no longer feels they are needed as much as they were in the past. The person may feel ground down by life stressors. Thinking can become extreme and unhelpful, with the person having negative thoughts about themselves, their current situation and the future (Beck's so-called *negative cognitive triad*). They may see their situation as hopeless and feel helpless about it.

A range of physical symptoms can occur such as changes in sleep patterns and appetite (both increased and decreased) and reduced concentration. The person may experience increased pain in existing conditions exacerbated by their mood, or physical complaints such as headaches and digestive problems that may not respond well to analgesics or other medications such as antacids. Often the physical symptoms are the last thing to improve, and the first symptoms to reoccur during relapse.

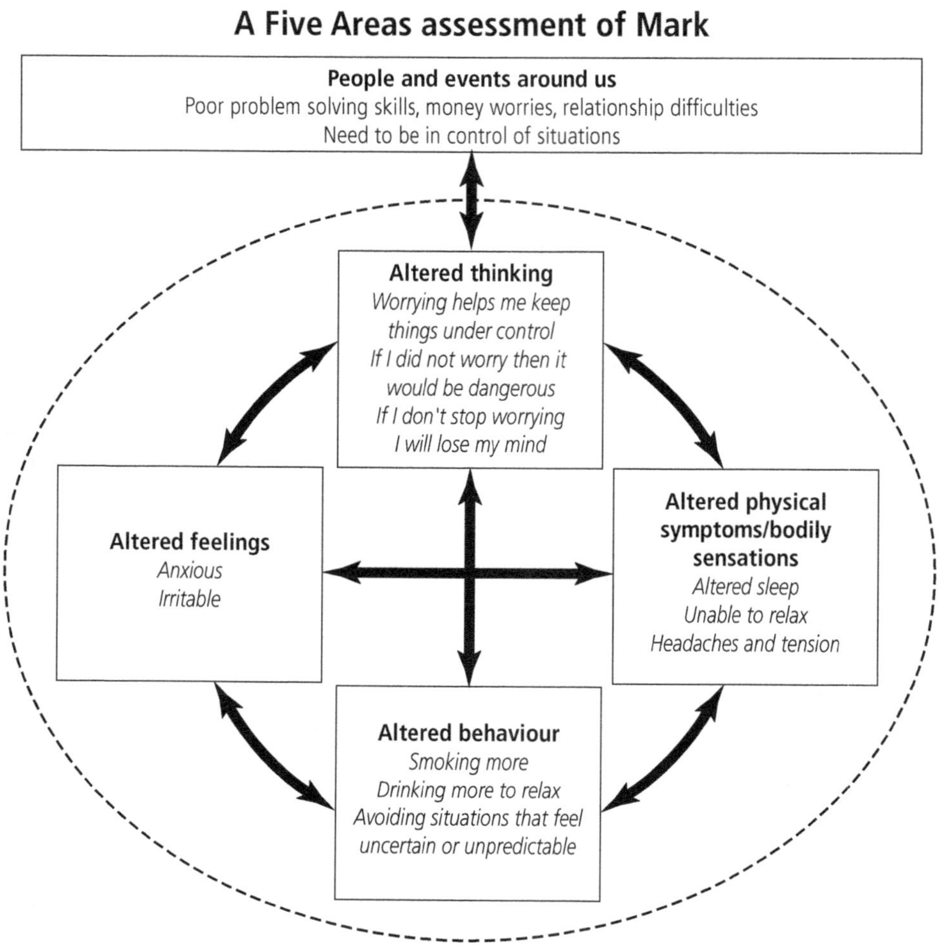

Figure 3.2 A Five Areas assessment of Mark, who has generalised anxiety.

Behaviour changes are common, with a reduction in activity and not attending to necessary tasks, leading to further deterioration in mood. In other words, there are vicious circles of reduced activity (with reduced pleasure, sense of achievement and closeness to others) and unhelpful behaviours. This is illustrated in Figure 3.3.

Panic disorder

In panic disorder the person catastrophically misinterprets internal symptoms (the physical symptoms of anxiety they get) as a sign of imminent harm or danger. Catastrophic fears boost the feelings of fear. For example, the patient whose legs shake may interpret this as a sign that they will collapse, a person who experiences pins and needles or an increased heart rate may interpret this as a sign that they are having a stroke, and the person whose mouth goes dry may misinterpret this as a sign that they are going to choke or suffocate. During a panic attack there is intense fear (panic) which peaks rapidly and usually only lasts a short time (20–40 minutes maximum).

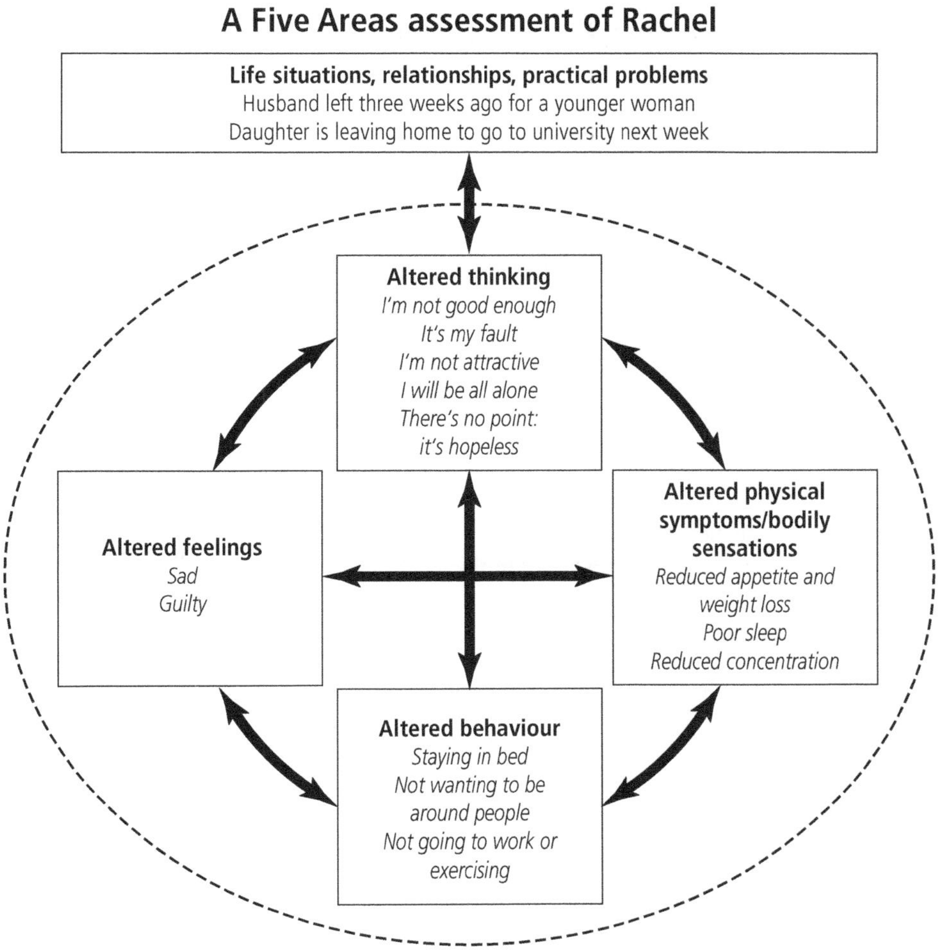

Figure 3.3 A Five Areas assessment of Rachel, who is feeling low.

Behaviours that aim to help the person feel safer (so-called *safety behaviours*) and avoidances result from the fears. So, the person with a dry mouth may carry bottled water, the person with wobbly legs may sit down if they feel they are getting anxious, and the person who experiences pins and needles or an increased heart rate may avoid situations where their heart rate could rise, such as climbing stairs, exercise or enjoying sex. They then mistakenly come to believe that their worst feared consequence did not occur simply because they carried out the safety behaviour. These behaviours are then repeated again and again, leading to undermined confidence in their own ability to cope and a restricted life as a result of the increasing avoidance.

Figure 3.4 illustrates how panic disorder can take over a person's life.

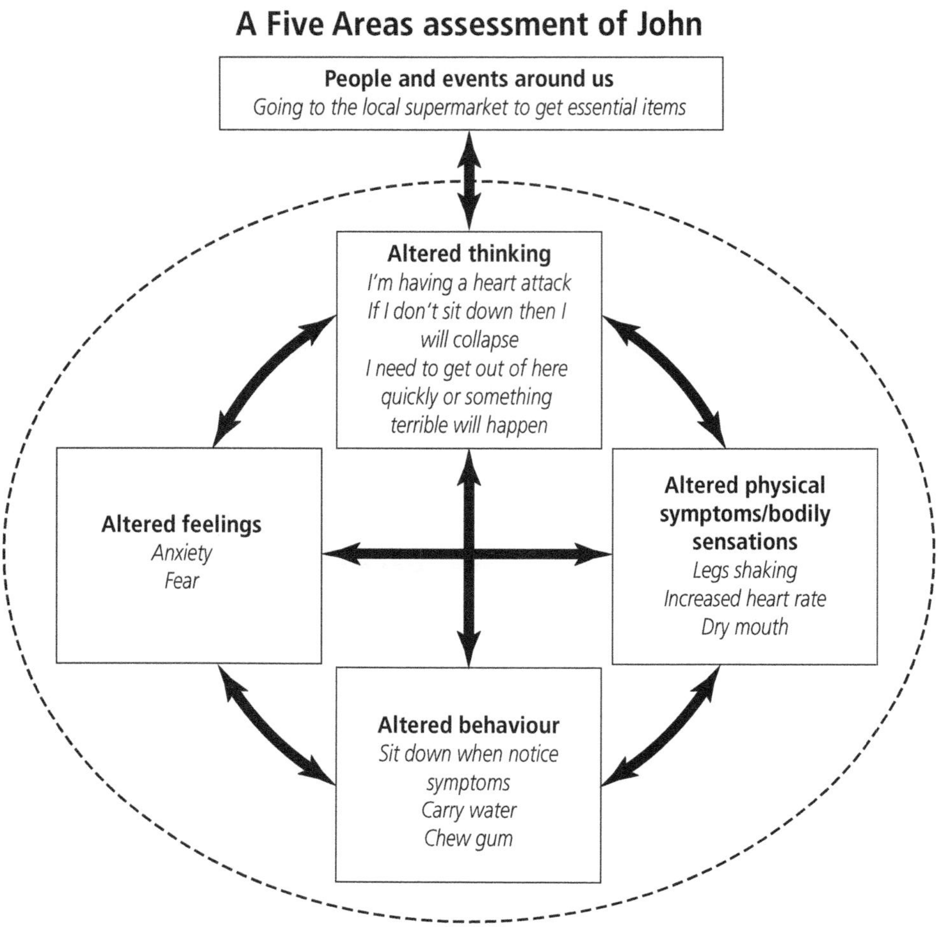

Figure 3.4 A Five Areas assessment of John, who experiences panic when going to the supermarket.

Obsessive compulsive disorder

A theme in obsessive compulsive disorder (OCD) is an over-estimation of harm occurring to the person or to others and a heightened sense of responsibility for that harm. So, for example, the person may experience unpleasant fears of their partner being in an accident, or may feel compelled to carry out a compulsive activity, such as repeatedly washing their hands or checking on something again and again or carrying out other rituals (behaviours) to neutralise the fear they feel as a result of the thought or image. The altered feelings are anxiety focused, with linked bodily arousal that reflects the level of fear experienced. Although the person experiences the thoughts as 'repugnant' and does not wish to have them, they still feel a compulsion to carry out the behaviour, even if they do not wish to do so.

Since acting in this way does make people with OCD feel less anxious, such checking behaviours quickly become established. The patient will feel scared if asked to reduce or stop the behaviours. More and more of life is taken over by the rituals or hidden mental equivalents such as counting a set number of times, saying 'It's okay' repeatedly, or praying obsessively.

Avoidance and safety behaviours unique to the patient can be quite subtle so a thorough assessment is needed.

Figure 3.5 summarises the affect of OCD on a person's life.

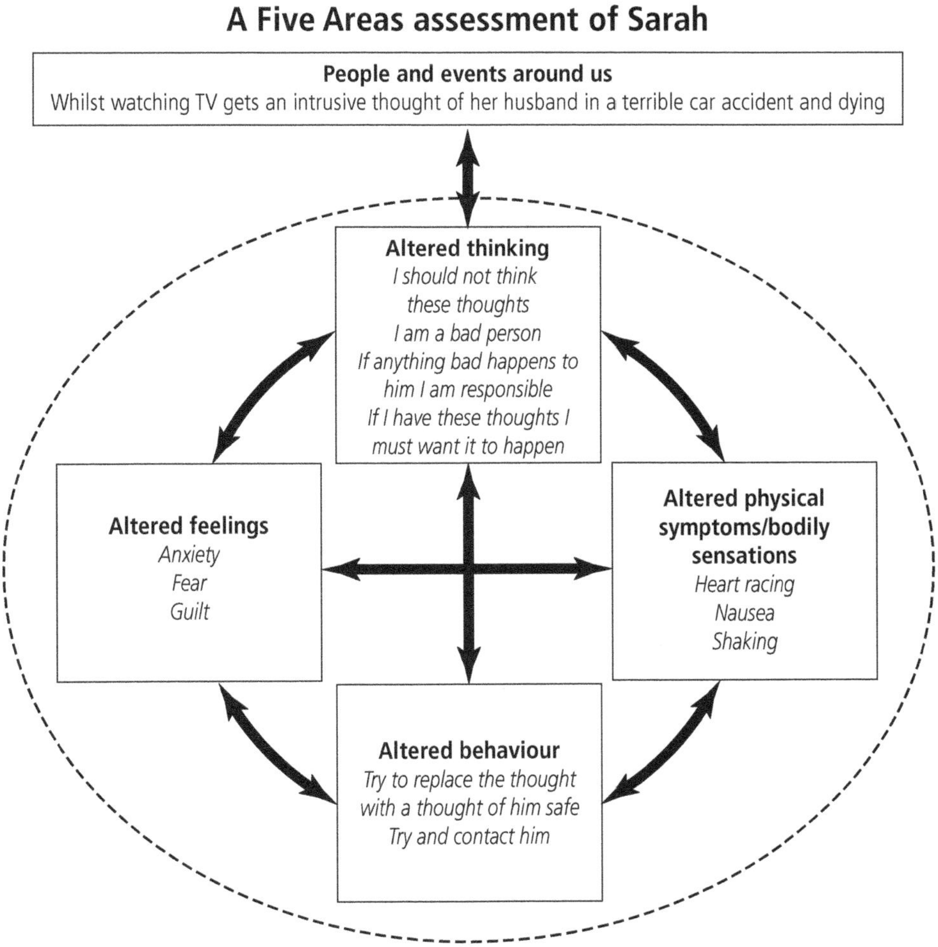

Figure 3.5 A Five Areas assessment of Sarah, who has obsessive compulsive disorder.

Health anxiety

The person with health anxiety (also known as hypochondriasis) has a fear of having a particular illness or disease, and misinterprets physical symptoms as a sign that confirms that illness. In panic the fear might be of collapsing *right now*, whereas in health anxiety the fear is of significant and nasty illness that will cause harm or damage to the person *at some time in the future*. It is important to confirm the diagnosis of health anxiety with a proper physical history and appropriate investigations, as many physical disorders also cause anxiety-style presentations (such as heart disease, asthma, thyroid dysfunction, chest or heart diseases and diabetes). Do not fall into the trap of making a premature and incorrect 'psychological' diagnosis when the problem has a physical cause. Referral to the patient's general practitioner or other practitioner to establish what is and what isn't present physically can therefore be helpful.

In health anxiety, anxiety is predominant. The anxious concerns lead to physiological arousal, and selective attention focused on the person's own body, which is then misinterpreted as evidence of the illness. The same occurs with common everyday bodily sensations and also symptoms of mild but self-limiting diseases such as colds and tummy bugs. For example, a person may have health anxiety related to a brain tumour, and may misinterpret eye strain or headaches as a sign that they have a tumour.

Patients with health anxiety are likely to seek repeated consultation with health professionals, and some may even have had exploratory tests or treatment. Often a number of practitioners are seen in various specialties in various hospitals. False positive results of investigations reinforce fears.

Safety behaviours such as presenting and re-presenting to health professionals for further tests and reassurance only reduce anxiety for a short time before the person seeks even more tests and still more reassurance. Again, avoidances and safety behaviours unique to the person should be assessed thoroughly. For example the person with health anxiety of a brain tumour may take medication for pain relief as a preventive measure so as not to experience a headache.

Figure 3.6 illustrates how health anxiety can affect the five areas.

Specific phobias

People with a specific phobia have anxiety related to a specific situation or object, such as a fear of flying, needles, blood, or a particular animal or insect. The specific object or situation is perceived as an overestimated threat of harm to the person, and this perception leads to avoidances and safety seeking behaviours in relation to situations or places where they may come into contact with the feared stimulus.

Emotional and physical changes during phobias are similar to panic, as are the range of avoidance, reassurance seeking and checking behaviours that occur. People can end up leading highly impaired and restricted lives.

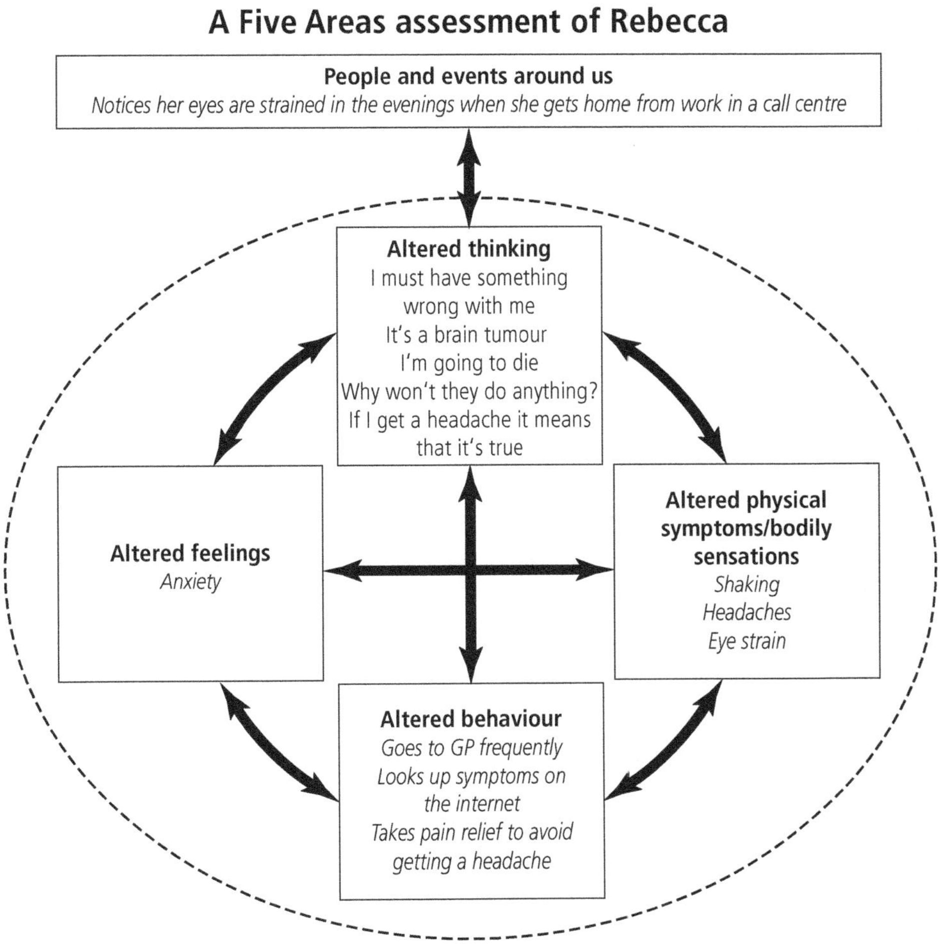

Figure 3.6 A Five Areas assessment of Rebecca, who has health anxiety.

Blood and injury phobias (including needles) are the only anxiety disorder in which the person may faint. For a person to faint, a rapid reduction in blood pressure has to happen. When a person is anxious during a panic attack, generally blood pressure increases rapidly and there is no possibility of a faint. In contrast, in blood and injury phobias blood pressure actually drops, so it makes evolutionary sense for the person to fall or lie down, so that the head and heart are on the same vertical level, thereby maximising blood flow to the brain (the so-called vasovagal response).

A specific phobia is illustrated in Figure 3.7.

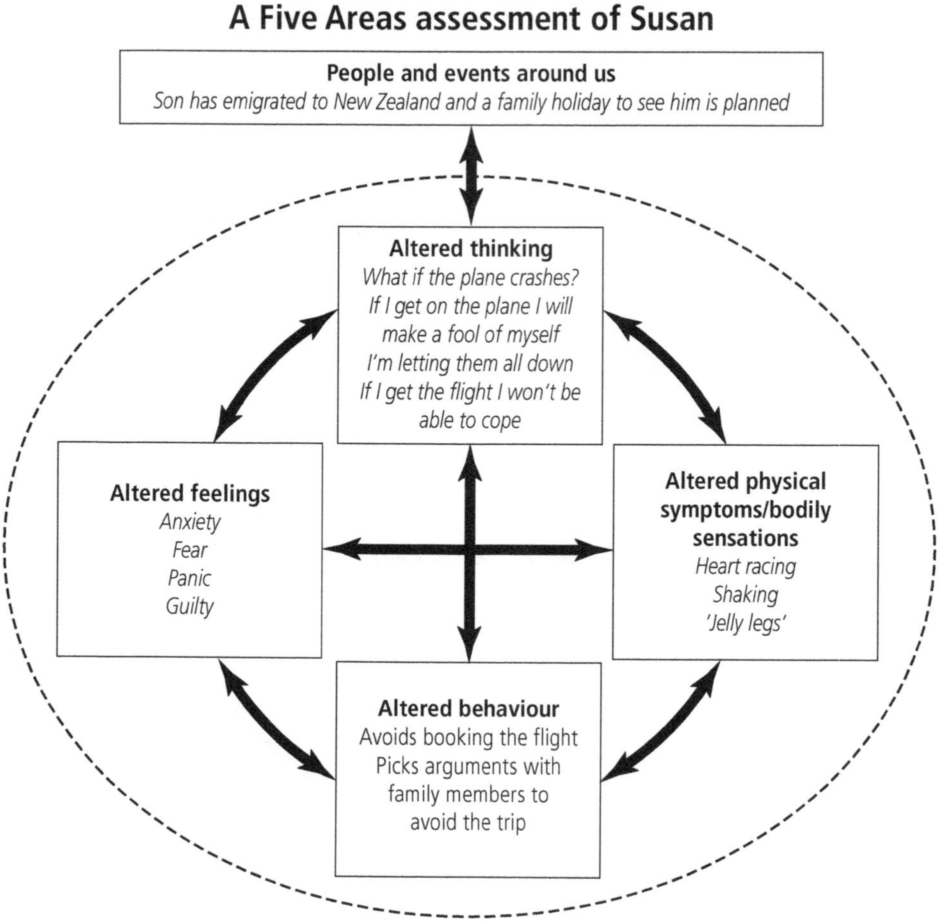

Figure 3.7 A Five Areas assessment of Susan, who has a phobia of flying.

Schizophrenia

In schizophrenia, paranoid beliefs and delusions can lead to understandable fears and resulting behaviours. So, for example, someone with a fear that spies are following or filming them with a view to abducting and torturing them (beliefs) might feel fearful, and notice physiological arousal when fearful (e.g. breathing faster and not sleeping well). They may alter their behaviour with avoidance (e.g. of going out alone) and safety behaviours (such as adding an extra lock to the door).

People with schizophrenia may understandably respond unhelpfully to their fears. So, they may make accusations against neighbours, carry a concealed knife, and sleep in their clothes in case they have to flee. They may hear voices (auditory hallucinations) that seem entirely real. One situation we have sometimes used to illustrate this to students involves recording surprising or critical statements on to an MP3 player. This is then played through headphones while we carry out a conversation with the student. They invariably appear vacant, disconnected (because their focus is elsewhere) and vague. This reinforces to them how distracting it is for the person with schizophrenia experiencing hallucinations.

The Five Areas model can helpfully be used with the patient (during recovery) and carers (with the patient's consent) to help explain why they are feeling and acting as they are. In higher intensity settings, it also provides a useful way of identifying areas of avoidance and isolation that may be good targets for change.

Figure 3.8 shows how schizophrenia can affect a person's life.

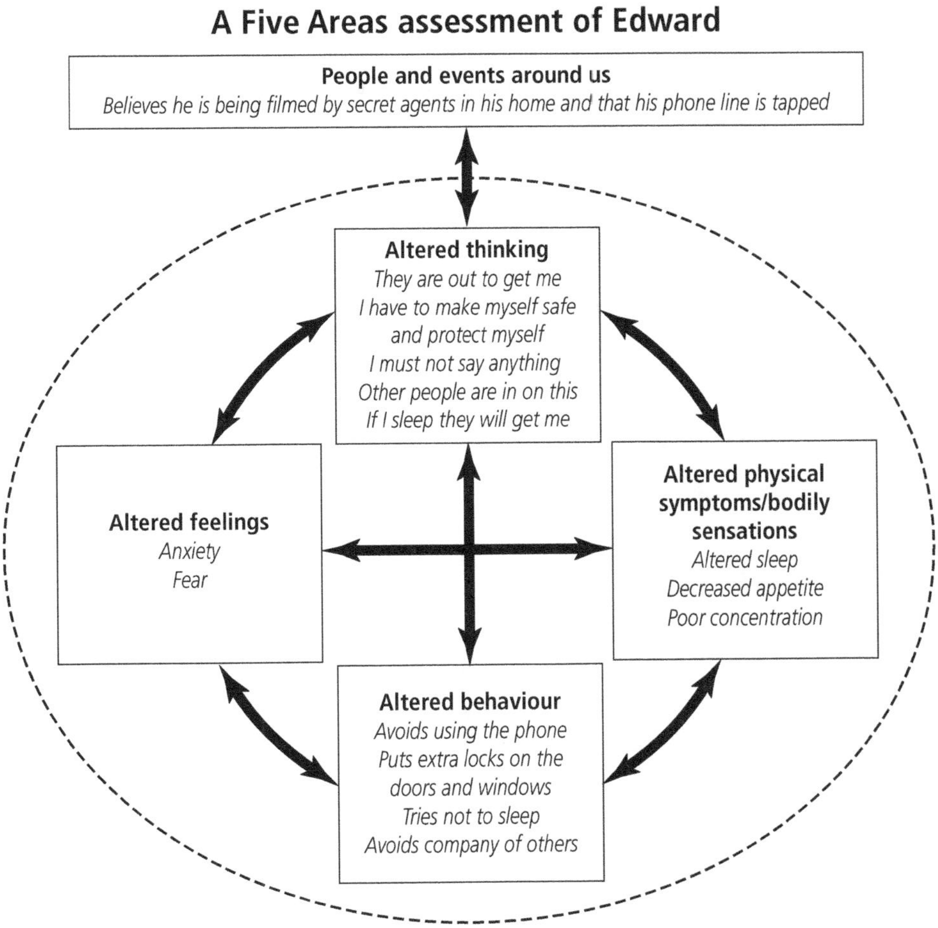

Figure 3.8 A Five Areas assessment of Edward, who has paranoid beliefs.

Dementia

In dementia, the person becomes progressively more disoriented in terms of time, place and person. Short-term memory is classically impaired, so the person with dementia finds it difficult forming new memories, while their long-term memory of events in their youth may be remarkably well preserved. They may lose weight because of poor appetite, and become prone to chest infections. Other physical symptoms (e.g. because of stroke) may be present. Their behaviour can reflect their confusion, with night-time wandering, problems getting dressed, getting lost when outside, and also misunderstandings of where they are or who they are with. These misunderstandings explain some of the emotional changes (depression, fear, hostility) that occur in dementia, and also can helpfully provide an overview of what is happening for carers.

Figure 3.9 summarises the Five Areas assessment of a person with dementia.

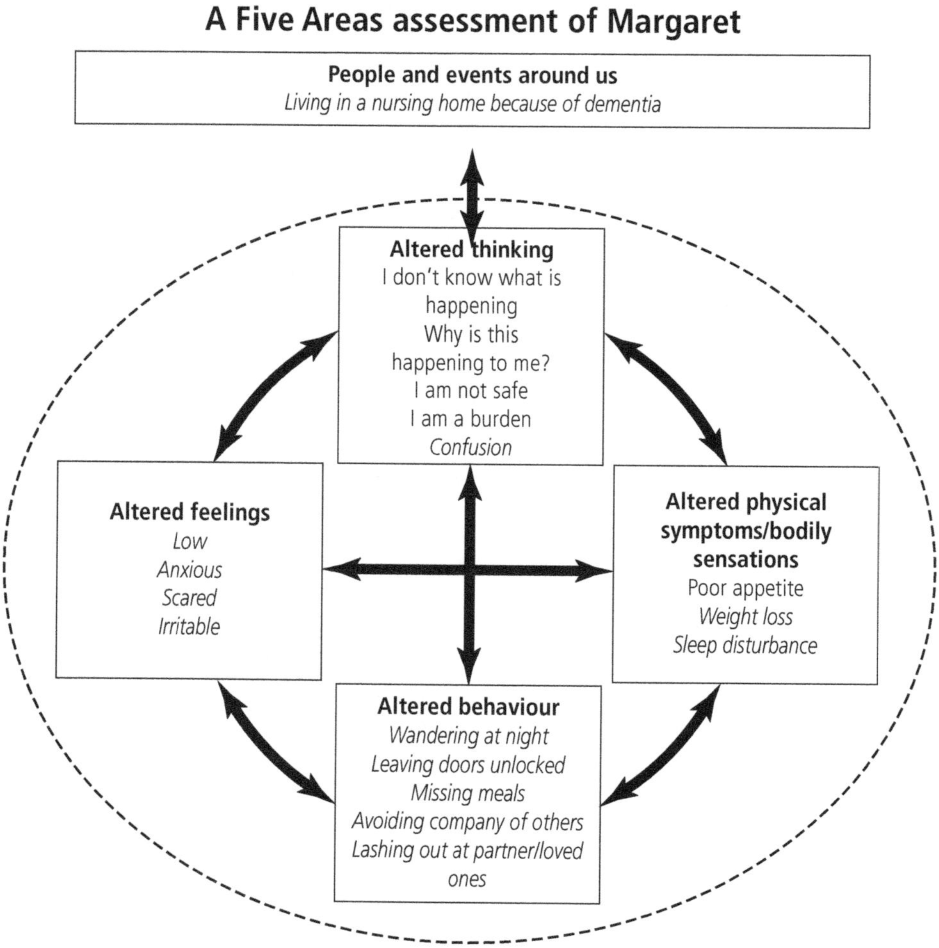

Figure 3.9 A Five Areas assessment of Margaret, who has dementia.

Key symptoms in different physical health disorders

The Five Areas assessment is not just relevant to mental health disorders. It is an integrated approach that can be flexibly applied across a range of disorders, for example in pain and with other long-term conditions. The following example illustrates how the approach can be used to help people make sense of physical symptoms and their impact.

Long-term pain, e.g. arthritis and chronic fatigue

Pain is not usually experienced as a pleasant thing. Chronic pain can be terrible, disabling and a focus of unhelpful thinking. Catastrophic predictions of the pain worsening, of not coping and of hopelessness may occur. A lack of knowledge of anatomy and how the body works leaves plenty of scope for misunderstanding information, and for having inaccurate fears about the impact of disease. Selective attention on swollen and painful joints and anxiety can worsen the perception of pain. Consequently, behaviour can be altered unhelpfully with reduced activity.

For many pain conditions, such as low back pain, keeping active is important. A doctor's advice needs to be sought about when rest is important, but beyond the acute phase of inflammation usually paced activity is the best way forward. Pain killers can be used inappropriately or in excess. A boom–bust vicious circle can occur where people do too much on a day with less pain, leading to tiredness and exhaustion and an increase of pain, which then negatively affects activity levels and what the person can do in the coming days.

Figure 3.10 shows an example of using the Five Areas assessment model for a person with pain.

Many people with long-term conditions can feel demoralised and ground down by symptoms. Chronic symptoms cause frustration and anger, and can result in depression and anxiety. The symptoms themselves can make the patient feel ill – and this can be worsened by added symptoms due to low mood or stress. Regardless of whether symptoms have a clear cause in terms of the presence of disease (such as arthritis, heart disease or asthma) or have not as yet been clearly identified (such as in chronic fatigue syndrome), there are helpful CBT interventions that can help the patient cope with symptoms.

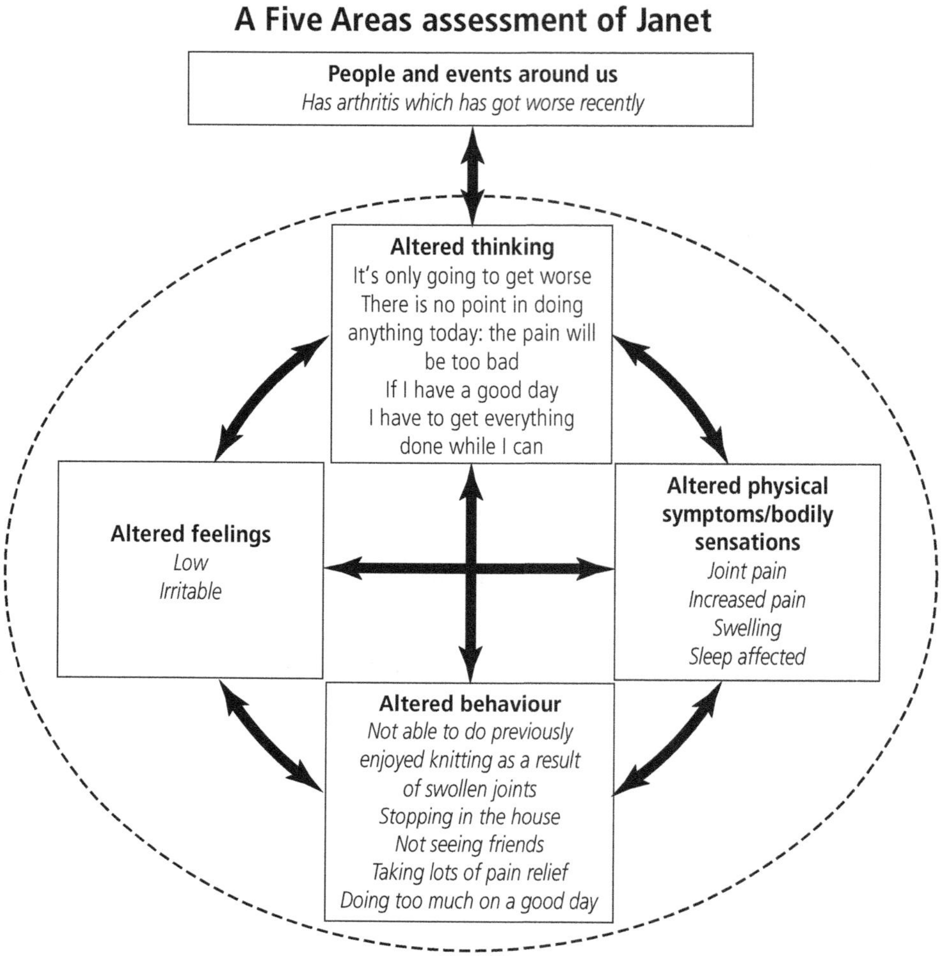

Figure 3.10 A Five Areas assessment of Janet, who has arthritis.

Carer responses

Research has shown time and time again that it is not easy to be a carer. There may be worrying thoughts and concerns about the patient being cared for. The carer may feel anxious, depressed or unable to cope as they try to offer support. Sometimes they may feel let down by the person who is ill, or they may get angry and resentful. These symptoms are associated with a range of anxiety, anger and depression-linked physical responses.

Sometimes stress leads to ongoing but unhappy relationships with anger, shouting, criticism and occasionally violence. Some carers find things so difficult that they leave home – possibly resulting in a total breakdown of relationships, e.g. divorce. Crucially, altered behaviour can worsen not only how the carer feels (e.g. drinking heavily) but also the patient they are supporting and caring for. This manifests itself in two key ways:

- **A high number of critical comments and a hostile approach to the patient**. This may be the result of frustration and anger aimed at the person. For example, in anorexia it is not uncommon for parents to shout, lock their child in the dining room or sometimes even attempt to force-feed their child. These actions backfire, with loss of trust, causing more anger and worsening the situation. Work here needs to focus on learning new skills to assertively encourage eating without loss of temper.
- **Emotional over-involvement**. A second common way that caring behaviour can backfire is when carers show their love by trying to wrap the patient in cotton wool. They take over all responsibility for everything. This may lead the carer to do everything for the patient, even answering on their behalf when the patient is asked a question. Such behaviour patterns can be frustrating for the patient, undermine confidence, and cause upset and anger.

Further information

Workbooks for carers to help them offer the best kind of support are included in the *Overcoming depression and low mood* book and *Overcoming teenage low mood and depression* book.

www.overcominganorexiaonline.com is an online resource aimed at family and friends of people with anorexia. It has been shown to reduce high expressed emotion, help carers be less depressed and anxious, and reduce negative care giving.

Key practice points

- Different disorders may cause disorder-specific patterns in each of the five areas and themes and typical behaviour changes can help to identify these correctly.
- Establishing a trusting therapeutic relationship is the core factor underpinning effective working.
- Verbal and non-verbal 'common factors' are very important in building a therapeutic relationship with the patient.

Further reading

Williams CJ, Garland A. (2002) A cognitive behavioural therapy assessment model for use in everyday clinical practice. *Advances in Psychiatric Treatment* **8**: 172–9. Available at: http://apt.rcpsych.org/cgi/reprint/8/3/172.

Wright B, Williams C, Garland A. (2002) Using the five areas cognitive-behavioural therapy model with psychiatric patients. *Advances in Psychiatric Treatment* **8**: 307–15. Available at: http://apt.rcpsych.org/cgi/reprint/8/4/307.

Chapter 4

Using the Five Areas assessment to understand why the person feels as they do

What you will learn

In this chapter you will learn how to complete a collaborative Five Areas assessment focused on how the person responds at the specific times when they feel worse. This acts as a working formulation of the current difficulties faced by the person in each of the five areas. The chapter will cover how to:

- Use the Five Areas assessment to understand why the person currently feels the way they do.
- Identify useful questions to ask in carrying out a Five Areas assessment, and why they are important.
- Look at ways of helping the person understand the links between the different areas.
- Boost engagement– and introduce the possibility of change.

Other linked chapters are Chapter 5, which covers how to choose a first (and subsequent) target for change, and Chapter 6, which covers how to provide support in using the Five Areas resources to facilitate this change.

Key Point

The assessment described here is appropriate for the 30–60-minute assessment time available to some practitioners. For shorter assessment times more of the Five Areas assessment would be focused on the patient completing this whole assessment using the written or online method of self-assessment as described in Chapter 3, which could be supplemented by a short review of specific times when the patient has felt worse.

The Five Areas assessment

As discussed in Chapter 3, the Five Areas assessment model is a pragmatic, structured process in which the patient's presenting problems and difficulties are summarised and broken down into key interlinked areas.

Area 1: *People and events* around the person. In other words, this examines the different *life situations, relationships* (supportive or not), *practical problems and personal resources* available to the patient.

Area 2: *Altered thinking*. Thinking can become extreme and unhelpful. Such thoughts are more frequent and become harder to deal with than usual, and worsen how the person feels or unhelpfully alter what they do when they feel distressed.

Area 3: *Altered emotions/feelings*. The person may have more than one altered mood. So, for example, when a person is feeling low or anxious they may also become irritable or distressed, and feel angry or ashamed at various times. The main emotional states are *happiness*, *sadness*, *anxiety*, *love*, *guilt*, *shame*, *fear* and *anger*. When distressed, a person may experience a range of these emotions. The cognitive behavioural therapy (CBT) approach uses such altered emotions as a way of identifying changes in underlying thinking.

Area 4: *Altered physical symptoms*. Physical symptoms can occur as a result of emotional change (e.g. biological symptoms of depression, somatic arousal in anxiety), or can be the result of an existing health condition such as diabetes, airways disease or coronary heart disease. **Note**: pain may be worse during anxiety and depression and may not respond as well to analgesics.

Area 5: *Altered behaviour or activity levels*. When changes in the four areas described above build up, it is to be expected that the patient will struggle to live their life as usual. They may alter what they do either helpfully and/or unhelpfully. They may do less of the things they previously enjoyed and *reduce their activity*, or may *avoid* things when anxious leading to restrictions in their daily life. People may also start doing *unhelpful behaviours* that they didn't do before, such as seeking reassurance from others, drinking excessively or using illicit drugs to cope with how they are feeling. Importantly, they may also do *helpful activities* such as pacing things, meeting others and seeking appropriate help.

✓ Practical hints and tips

An example of the everyday use of the Five Areas approach is available on the Living Life to the Full website (**www.livinglifetothefull.com** or **www.llttf.com**) and on the LLTTF DVD. This uses the example of a person walking down the street and past someone they know, who doesn't say anything to them. They jump to the conclusion that the other person doesn't like them and feel worse. The example then shows another scenario: that perhaps the other person just didn't see them. It displays the model visually with symbols to represent each of the areas, as shown in Figure 4.1. Try to watch this clip while working through this chapter to aid understanding how thoughts, feelings and behaviour all act together to make the person feel worse and how to communicate this model to a patient.

Using the Five Areas assessment

The Five Areas assessment can be used to summarise:

- A specific time when the patient felt worse (or better) as described in the current chapter.
- Or as a general summary of their overall difficulties (as summarised in Chapter 3).

Task

A good way for practitioners to familiarise themselves with the Five Areas model is by carrying out their own Five Areas summary of a time when their own mood was altered. The practitioner should think back to a recent time when there was a noticeable change in their emotional state. They should choose a time or event that led them to feel **moderately upset**, for example an argument with a partner or a vehicle cutting them up when they were driving, or perhaps feeling down about something like not getting a job they had applied for. Do not choose something that led to very high or distressing emotions.

Next, the practitioner should imagine that situation again as if it was happening right now, 'live'– like they were replaying a DVD of the situation over in their mind. The practitioner should stop, think and reflect as they go through the five different areas that can be affected. Use the blank Five Areas diagram in Figure 4.1 on page 62.

Some issues to consider in completing a Five Areas assessment

The following are some issues that can cause confusion when completing a Five Areas assessment.

Differentiating between thoughts and feelings

When completing a Five Areas assessment, people can sometimes get confused about which symptoms to put in which box. This is partly because of the way the English language is, which sometimes confuses thoughts and emotions.

✓ Practical hints and tips

The way the words 'I feel' are used can cause confusion. For example, is 'I feel like going to the shops' a thought or a feeling? Which area of the diagram do you think this belongs in? It is in fact a thought or opinion – not an emotion – I am considering going to the shops.

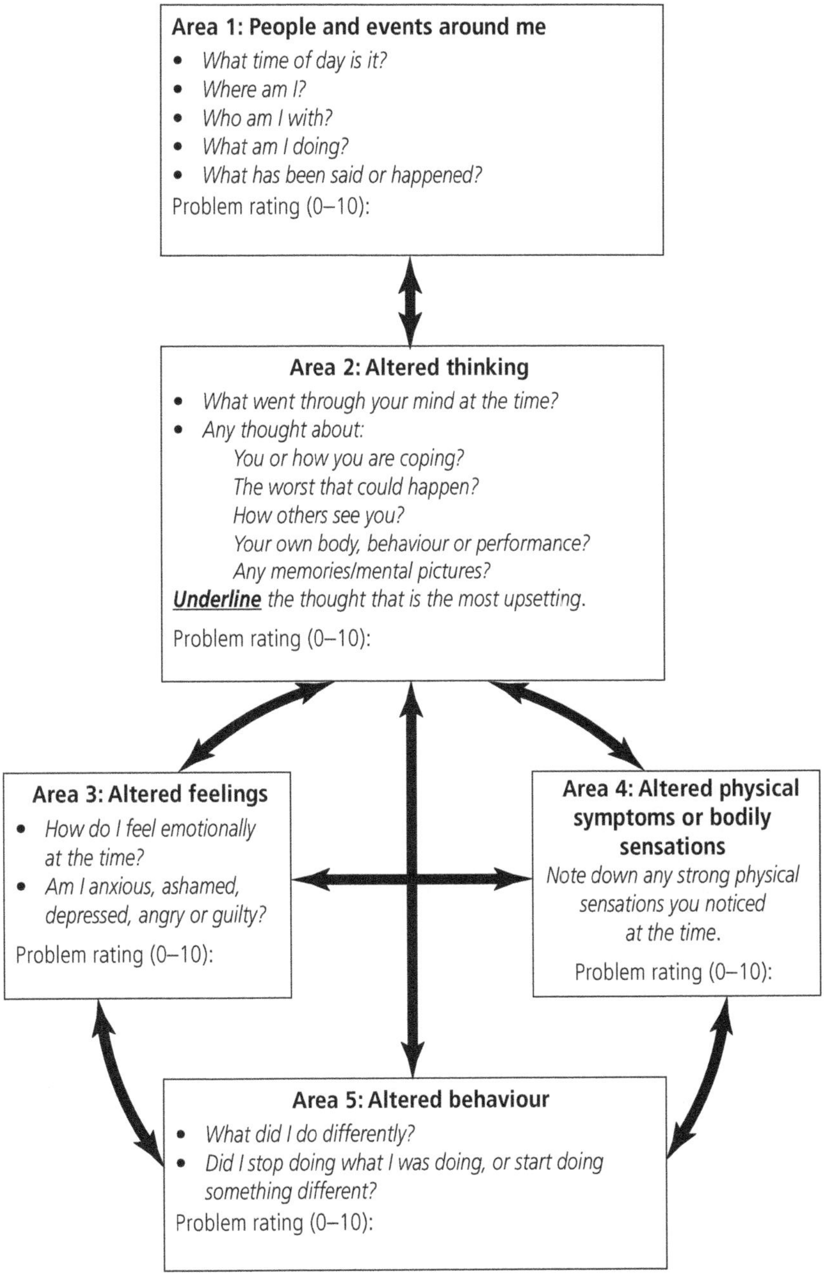

Figure 4.1 Summary of the practitioner's own Five Areas assessment of a time when they felt mild to moderately worse.

Task

Decide which of the following are thoughts and which are emotions:

	Tick here if you think this is a thought	Tick here if you think this is a emotion
1. I feel angry		
2. I feel so fed up		
3. I can't do anything		
4. I feel down		
5. Everyone hates me		
6. I'm blazing mad		
7. I feel so useless		
8. I feel pxxxxx off!		
9. I'm worried about my job		
10. I feel so ashamed		
11. I feel confused		

(Answers: 1, 2, 4, 6, 8, 10 are emotions, and 3, 5, 7, 9 and 11 are thoughts.)

Metaphors and the language of emotion

Many people use metaphors to describe emotions. For example, depression is often described as feeling blue/flat/grey/empty or like being under a black cloud. Sir Winston Churchill used to describe his depression as his 'black dog'. Anxiety is often called 'nerves' and stress can be used to describe both low mood and anxiety, so it is important to check what the patient means when using certain words so the practitioner has the right understanding. As long as the practitioner can make the link to the emotion they are describing, it is useful and beneficial to the patient to use their own words and language in the assessment and on the summary diagram.

The language of emotion and physical symptoms

Sometimes the patient (for whatever reason, e.g. habit, learned in their family of origin, a reaction to stigma, cultural reasons or out of personal preference) seems to communicate emotional distress using a language of physical symptoms rather than using a language of emotions. So, someone who appears anxious or down might instead say 'I'm tired' or 'It hurts' rather than saying that they feel distressed. Very often people feel uncomfortable and reject mental health labels such as anxiety and depression.

The danger is that if a mental health professional insists on using mental health words (such as depression), the patient will disengage and drop out. It's a bit like someone who speaks French trying to communicate with someone who speaks Spanish. Both can understand some words spoken by each other, but key concepts could still be completely misunderstood.

A useful approach here again is to use the patient's own words. The impact of symptoms can be slowly introduced by using non-emotional concepts such as 'It must be frustrating not being able to do the things you want', or 'All these things can build up to really grind anyone down'. Most people find such terms acceptable and are happy to think of themselves in these ways. If the patient feels strongly, cross out the words 'Altered feelings/ emotions' in that box and swap it for something like 'Impact on me'.

Another common situation is when a patient describes themselves as feeling 'terrible' rather than a more recognisable word such as depressed. Here, the practitioner could ask, 'When you felt terrible like that, where were you?' or 'How did you feel in your body when you felt terrible like that?' or 'So when you were feeling terrible, were you aware of any emotional changes at the time?', etc.

Questions to ask the patient to get the required information

When training practitioners in clinical assessment skills, one of the most frequently asked question we encounter is 'What should I be asking to get the information I need?' This is understandably a concern, because a clinician undertaking an assessment has to bear many things in mind at once. The first step is to put the patient at ease as much as possible. The practitioner can try putting themselves in the patient's shoes and imagine how they might be feeling. An introductory chat before beginning the main assessment can help to do this. For example, ask if the patient found the place easily. The next section discusses this in more detail.

Consider what may be going through the patient's mind. They may be thinking that the practitioner will judge them in some way, or that being referred to a mental health practitioner is a sign of weakness as they haven't managed to sort their problems out by themselves. All of these thoughts can impact on engagement.

Thus the questions that are asked should be structured and have the overall aim of working towards a shared understanding of the patient's Five Areas summary diagram.

How to conduct a collaborative Five Areas assessment

Introduction to the assessment

> ✔ **Practical hints and tips**
>
> Don't spend a lot of time in this section going through in detail all the treatments that the service may offer the patient. Remember they haven't been assessed yet, and some interventions may not be suitable for their difficulties or acceptable to them at this point. They may require referral to another practitioner at a higher step of care. So the practitioner may be offering something they can't guarantee that they could actually have. It is much preferred to leave the discussion of possible treatment options until the end of the assessment when the practitioner and the patient have a clearer understanding of the presenting problem.
>
> Similarly, the practitioner would not want to send out too much information or self-help resources in the post to a patient in advance of the initial assessment appointment as this can seem overwhelming.

The introduction is probably one of the most important parts of the assessment process, and sometimes the least well thought through. A good practitioner will put the patient at ease and explain what is going to happen.

The process to follow is given below.

1) **Introduce yourself, check the patient's full name and what they would like to be called** and make a note of this. They may have an abbreviated name they prefer to use, or use their middle name.

   Give your full name, and tell the patient how you would like to be addressed.

2) **Explain your role**, remembering that this is unlikely to mean much to the patient, **so say what you do**. For example: 'I am a wellbeing coach, and what this means is that I have received training to provide support and guidance to people with problems such as low mood or anxiety.'

3) To set the scene, inform the patient that the **purpose** of the session is a **collaborative assessment** to see if the interventions you can provide may be helpful for their current difficulties. This allows the patient to consider if this is something they might be interested in taking forward.

4) Tell them the **amount of time** the assessment will take and ask whether this time is okay for them. They may not have realised how long it will take and have to leave early or alter their transport plans.

5) Explain that the **assessment is structured**: that you will begin by asking them to talk about a recent example of their current difficulties, the impact these are having on their daily life and how they may have developed, to work out if any particular behaviours might be worsening the situation.

6) Let the patient know that you will be **asking lots of questions**, and at times you may have to stop them and come back to things they have already said, so everything they say is important.

7) Tell them there will be some **time at the end** for anything else they feel hasn't been covered and for checking that you have understood their problem properly. (The patient may not have had a CBT-based assessment before and they may be expecting to come and 'tell their story' in a less structured way.)

8) Explain that everything they say is **confidential**. Be specific here: is this just between you and them, or will you need to share this information with your supervisor or other people within the team you work in, and with their own general practitioner?

9) Explain the **two exclusions to confidentiality**. If you believe that there is a *risk of harm to them or to another person* you would have to pass this on. You may want to give the patient an example here. Explain that if you were to tell anyone else, *you would try to inform them first*.

10) Explain that you will be **taking notes and how these will be used**. Will you be writing a report to the referrer or are they just for the notes within the service? Clarify if you are happy for the patient to have a copy of what you write, and if there are any processes to be followed in this case.

11) If you are using **standardised measures**, for example the Increasing Access to Psychological Therapies (IAPT) Minimum Data Set. Explain **why, when and how often this will be repeated**. Give the patient a clear understanding of the benefits of the measures **to them** and also how they will be used in the service.

12) Ask the patient if they have any **questions** before you begin, either about the process or about you. Clarify if it is okay for them to ask you questions as you go along if there is anything they do not understand or are unsure about.

Starting the assessment

Start the assessment by asking about the main problem the patient is having.

Q Can you describe in your own words what you see as your main problem currently?

Q Can you tell me how you are feeling currently in terms of numbers? Think that 0 per cent is the best you've ever felt and 100 per cent is the worst it has ever been for you.

Rating each of the five areas is important. It gives a baseline for comparisons in the future that is personal and specific to the patient. The self-help resources encourage the patient to self-rate the extent of their problems in each area.

Specific event summary

Next, focus on the specific times they have felt worse.

The aim of the specific example is to gather information about the patient's recent difficulties in each of the five areas, in the same way you did your own assessment earlier in the chapter. The specific example gives a personal example of the model in action that can be used at the end of the assessment to illustrate the links between thoughts, feelings, physical symptoms and altered behaviours. Should, for any reason, the assessment get interrupted, or not get finished (perhaps the practitioner wants to discuss the case with their supervisor before they discuss treatment options or make any decisions), talking about a specific event ensures that the model can be at least introduced to the patient and is informative and helpful to other professionals who may take on the case if it is stepped up or signposted elsewhere.

Going through a focused and specific time when the patient has felt worse also provides a record of how things were prior to starting treatment. This can be used as a baseline for assessment of progress during treatment. Patients often easily disregard their successes or forget where they were with the problem when they started. Having a written diagram summary and rating of the severity of symptoms in each of the five areas at the start of treatment is therefore very helpful.

✓ Practical hints and tips

Sometimes depressed patients struggle to recall a time when they have felt worse. This is understandable, given that the patient may feel depressed all or much of the time. The practitioner can do one of two things here: ask them to identify a time when they felt even just a little worse; or if there isn't a specific event they can recall, a good way of gathering specific information is to ask them to think about the previous day. The point of this is to have a baseline of how their low mood is affecting them during a 24-hour period. Then move straight to the impact section of the assessment (page 66).

Key questions to ask when carrying out the specific event summary

People and events (situations, relationships and practical problems)

Q

- Can you recall over the past few days when you have felt particularly low/sad/depressed/in pain? (Use the term the patient has used to describe themselves.)
- If yes, can you recall it as if it happening now, like you are watching a 'live' DVD of it in your mind?
- When was this?
- What time of day was it?
- Where were you?
- Who was with you, and what was going on around you?
- What was said?

Altered emotions/feelings

Q

- At what point in that specific situation did you feel most low/sad/depressed/in pain?
- Can you focus on that time as if it is happening now?
- Can you tell me what you were feeling emotionally and how strong that feeling was on a 0–10 scale, if 0 is not at all low/sad/depressed/in pain and 10 is the most low/sad/depressed/in pain you have ever felt?

Altered physical symptoms

Q

- When you were feeling the most upset, did you notice any physical symptoms in your body?
- How strong were those symptoms at that time? (Use the symptom that the patient described rather than just symptoms in general.)

Some patients can readily recall physical symptoms, but others may struggle. Often anxiety symptoms are recalled easily as they are quite unpleasant for the patient and may be misinterpreted as dangerous. For example, the anxious patient with a racing heart often thinks this is a sign of a heart attack, and then becomes panicky as a result.

Thoughts

- If you try to focus on the point that was most distressing in the situation for you, what was going through your mind at that point?
- Can you see any images or pictures in your mind?
- Did you have any thoughts about yourself or the situation at that time?
- How much did you believe that to be true at that time on a scale of 0–100 per cent?
- How much do you believe that to be true now on the same scale?

When asking about thoughts, note the question is not 'What thoughts did you have?' but is framed as 'What was going through your mind at that point?'. This includes images as well as verbal thoughts. For example, during a panic attack a patient may think they will collapse and then experience an image of an ambulance or of themselves on the floor with people gathered around them.

It is important to encourage the patient to focus on the situation as if it is happening right now. Thoughts are easier to recall if there is the emotional link to the situation. Images are also very important to ask about. Some people 'think' in images. For example, if you think about the happiest day of your life, do you get a picture in your mind or thoughts about the day, or both?

Altered behaviours

- At that specific time, what did you do as a result?
- Did you take any action to try to improve how you were feeling?
- How did you manage or try to cope with it?
- What do you think would have happened to you if you had not done that?
- How long did the feelings last (minutes, hours, days)?
- Was there anything that happened or didn't happen on that specific occasion that made it worse?

When asking about altered behaviour the aim is to see what they did differently as a result, which may have been helpful or may have unhelpfully backfired. Did they reduce their activity, add in unhelpful (safety) behaviours, or use strategies to feel better such as avoidance or escape?

- What made it go away?
- Is the event you have described a typical example of when you feel low/sad/depressed/in pain?

Summary of the specific event

The practitioner should summarise what the patient has said at this point to check their understanding of the patient's problem.

Example:

Harvinder comes to see a practitioner and says he had a difficult time this morning and felt 'terrible' when he went to the supermarket. The word 'terrible' describes the sum total of the whole impact on him of the situation. Break down what happened and take it slowly.

Practitioner: Where were you when you first started to feel terrible?

Harvinder: I was on my way to the supermarket and was getting quite close.

Practitioner: What time was it?

Harvinder: About 10.30 am.

(**Note**: *The practitioner asks other questions here to help get a clear idea of where Harvinder was, what he was doing and what else was going on.*)

Practitioner: What was the first thing you noticed?

(**Note**: *This is a good way of getting into the vicious circle.*)

Harvinder: I started to notice this tension in my shoulders ...

(**Note**: *The Five Areas is a vicious circle: it can start at any part of the circle and it doesn't always have to be a thought. Indeed in panic attacks quite often the first thing noticed is feeling physically unwell. The practitioner would ask more questions here to establish any other physical changes, and summarise it back to the patient.*)

Practitioner's summary statement: So, to start with you noticed tension in your shoulders, then you noticed your breathing speeding up, and a tight feeling in your chest and started to feel really unwell. Did you notice anything else then?... I wonder whether you noticed any change in how you felt emotionally when you felt unwell like that?

Harvinder: I'd been feeling a bit worried when I knew I had to get to the shops that morning – but I started to feel really scared just then with my chest getting tight and I began to breathe very fast.

Practitioner: So, you noticed a tight chest and speeded up breathing and tense shoulders, and you started to get really scared. How scared did you feel? Can you try to rate how you felt on the sheet here – you can see the scale of 0–10, where 0 is no problems at all and 10 is the worst you could possibly feel.

Harvinder: I'd have been about 6 or 7 to start with – I was feeling quite scared.

Practitioner: And what happened next?

A: My heart was thumping and as I entered the store my breathing speeded right up and my heart was really racing.

Practitioner: So, you were there with your heart really racing, your breathing speeded right up, feeling really scared – with a rating of 6 or 7 out of 10 for being scared. Did that scary feeling get any worse? (*Harvinder nods.*) Okay, how bad was that scary feeling when you felt at your very worst – again using the same scale?

Harvinder: I think it was heading for a 10 – more than a 10 – off the top of the scale.

Practitioner: What went through your mind at the time?

Harvinder: I don't remember. I just was aware of my breathing and feeling really bad.

Practitioner: So you were really focused on your breathing and feeling really bad. Were you aware at the time of what might happen if you couldn't calm your breathing? (*Harvinder nods.*) What was the worst that could happen?

Harvinder: That I was a goner – I'd be on the floor.

Practitioner: Before we move on to think about how you tried to cope, can we just talk a bit more about those fears: that you'd be on the floor and a goner. Which of those seemed the most scary thought?

Harvinder: I was sure **I was going to die** – that was it, I thought it was all over, I felt so bad.

Practitioner: It sounds like it was really difficult, and very scary. Let's try to understand even more about what was going on then. How much did you believe at the time you were going to die? Again, using this same 0–10 scale.

Harvinder: It was definitely a 10. I could see myself there on the floor.

Practitioner: So you were there – really convinced you were going to die – seeing yourself on the floor – you felt physically ill, you couldn't catch your breath. There was a lot going on. How did you try to cope with all this? How did you react?

Harvinder: Well earlier I tried to catch my breath, but it didn't work. I just felt like I was going to suffocate. I left the trolley and headed for the exit, I was almost running. I'll never go back there again.

Practitioner's summary statement: So now let's spend some time and try to work out step by step what happened. I've tried to write all the key things on this diagram. Let's talk it though together… So, to start with, you noticed tension in your shoulders, then you noticed your breathing speeding up, and a tight feeling in your chest and started to feel really unwell. You felt really scared – heading for a 10 – and saw yourself as a goner, on the floor, going to die – and that's when you left the trolley and headed for the exit running, and saying to me that you'll never go back there.

Harvinder: Yes, yes, that's right.

Practitioner: So now let me give you the pen, and let's see if there's anything you'd add here, or cross out? And also let's talk some more to try to work out how each of the five areas played a part in making things feel worse and worse at the time …

We are going to come back to think about this example later in this chapter (on page 71). However, before moving on, think about how the assessment is structured here. Consider how the practitioner has sequenced the questions. The replies use Harvinder's own words, contain a lot of summarising to check understanding – and slowly – with reference to the blank Five Areas diagram (which is filled in slowly at each stage), all five areas are systematically examined and discussed.

Note: How much time is spent discussing and understanding each of the areas will depend on how much time is available.

Why bother using the Five Areas assessment model?

Key Point

What is different with a CBT-based approach is the structure within which questions are asked. Often other forms of clinical assessment begin with finding out some history of the patient. The CBT-based Five Areas approach begins by the patient recollecting an example of how their current difficulties are affecting them in each of the five areas on a **recent occasion, i.e. here and now**. Then the impact the problem is having on the patient's daily life is assessed, and information is gathered about what may be maintaining the problem (keeping the problem going) and how it may have come about to see where an intervention may be possible.

The structured approach is a very important part of this process as the assessment should be collaborative and it should help the patient to begin to discover the links between the areas in which they are experiencing difficulty. This systematic approach is helpful for practitioners as it aids the understanding of the impact of depression or anxiety on the patient's subjective experience in each of the five areas, a set of inter-related problems rather than one large overwhelming problem. It also enables setting clear target areas for intervention.

Using the Five Areas summary diagram

Let's look at Harvinder's Five Areas summary in diagrammatic form (Figure 4.2)

The Five Areas diagram summary is repeatedly used during the assessment and should be visible to both the practitioner and the patient from time to time. In summarising back the model, the entire episode is talked through, following the time sequence the patient (Harvinder) described ('So first you noticed …'). As every new area is introduced, links can be made between the areas to help introduce the concept that each area can worsen each other as part of a vicious circle.

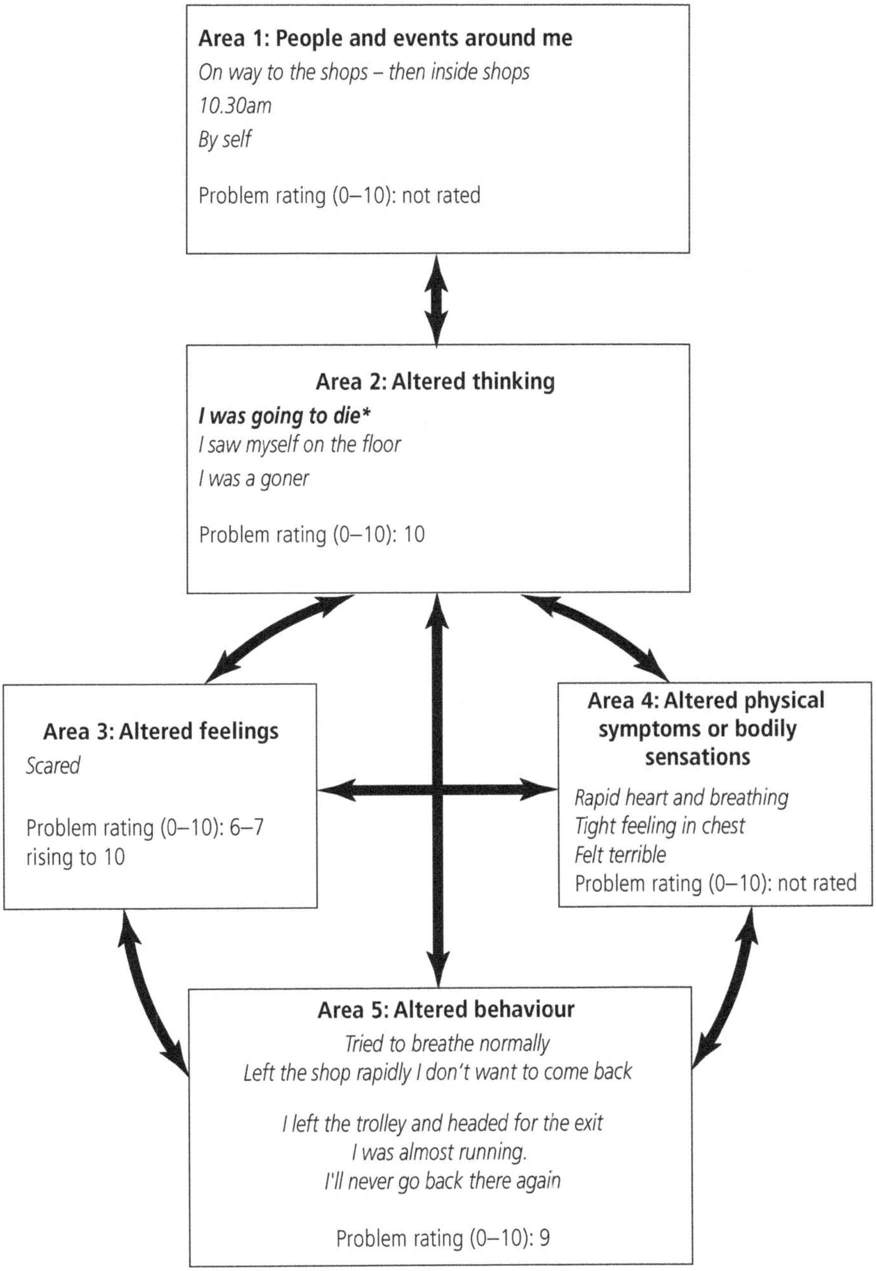

Figure 4.2 Harvinder's five areas summary.

Thought–feeling links

Q So, let's look at that time there on the diagram when you felt on the top of the scale of scared. How do you think believing those really scary thoughts fitted in with feeling scared like that?

Q If I had been in the same situation absolutely convinced I'm about to die right now, how do you think I might have felt?

Thought–behaviour links

Q So at that time you just knew you were going to die, and felt so bad emotionally and physically (*pointing to the boxes and arrows*). How do you think this all affected your decision to suddenly leave the shop just them?

Q Would it have made sense to keep shopping when you believed you were about to die at the time? How could you have found out what might have happened if you had stayed put?

The role of physical symptoms in worsening scary thoughts and emotions

Q Is it possible there are links between feeling so bad physically, as if you were suffocating, and feeling so scared?

Q Do you think anyone else in the same position and feeling so bad like that would have felt scared too?

There is an opportunity here for educating the patient about the fight or flight adrenaline response and how over-breathing makes people feel worse. The various Five Areas resources can be suggested as a way to provide this information between sessions.

Key Point

The main issue in the example is to help Harvinder realise that his thoughts, feelings, physical symptoms and behaviour changes can all be understood by him. His scary thoughts made him feel worse. When he felt more scared and physically ill, these symptoms reinforced his fears that he would die. It all built up and up and up until he felt he had to leave.

Q I just wondered, now we've gone through this, does it help you understand a bit more about what actually happened?

Linking this to the possibility of change

A key concept in the Five Areas model is that making changes in any one of these areas leads to change in other areas as well (this is a direct implication of the vicious circle model). The process of writing down their symptoms in this way is a helpful process for the patient, as it allows them to take a step back from what is happening and look at their situation more objectively – an outside-in perspective that can provide a degree of emotional distance from their experiences.

Ultimately, as mentioned in Chapter 1, the aim of the Five Areas assessment is a shared psychological understanding of the difficulties being experienced in each of the five areas, in an easy-to-use jargon-free CBT format. Have a go at summarising a patient whom you are currently seeing and supporting, or have seen in the past, using the diagram provided in Figure 4.3

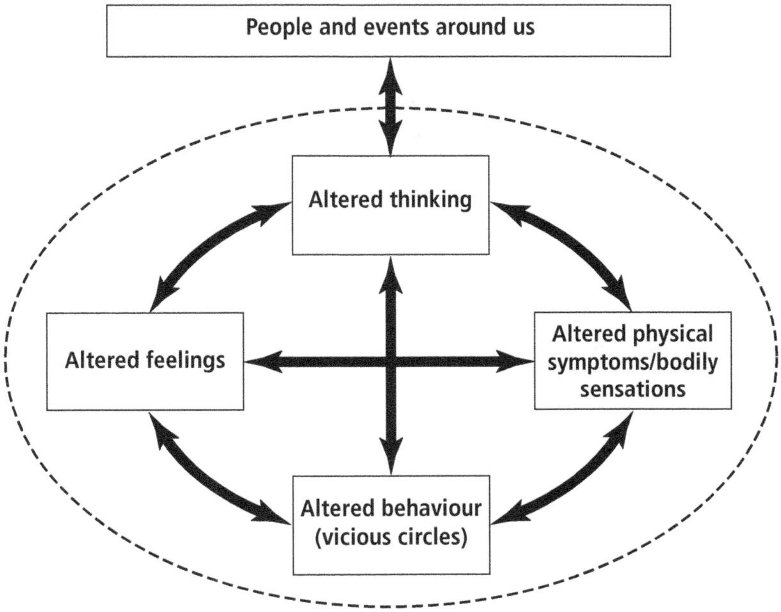

Figure 4.3 A Five Areas assessment summary of my patient.

Further exploration of the impact of the problem on daily life

Maintenance of the problem

After the initial assessment the practitioner can identify any areas of avoidance, reduced activity, etc. that are keeping the patient's symptoms going by asking the following questions.

Q

- Are there any other situations the patient associates with feeling worse?
- Are there any other situations that make them feel better?

- Have they noticed any triggers that make them feel worse?
- What are they not able to do as a result or are there any other places they cannot go as a result of this problem?
- Are there any things that they can do if someone is with them but they could not do alone?
- What do they predict would happen if they tried to do these things alone?
- Have they developed any strategies to help them avoid feeling anxious in these situations? (E.g. some people carry water in case their mouth gets dry or carry a mobile phone or medication with them, or avoid busy times at the supermarket.
- Would they be able to enter these situations without carrying out these things?
- Is there anything else they do to make themselves feel less anxious?
- Is there anywhere else they could not go as a result of feeling anxious?
- Do they drive?
- Are there places they will not drive as a result of feeling anxious?
- Can they use the motorway?
- If not, why not?
- What do they think could happen?

The questions about the maintenance of the problem alongside the questions asked about activities of daily living, alcohol and drug use and previously enjoyed activities give information about how behaviour has altered helpfully or unhelpfully as a result of the patient's current difficulties.

Helpful questions to assess the impact of a behaviour

What, Where, Why, When and with Whom questions

If avoidance or safety behaviours are identified, further enquiry should be made either during the assessment or prior to starting treatment on this area. The following questions can help explore these issues.

Q

- What can the patient do/not do as a result of anxiety?
- Why can they do the things they can do compared with the things they can't?
- What makes these things possible?
- Do they have coping strategies for these to reduce anxiety; for example, if they can go to the cinema do they have to sit on the end of the row so they can get out easily if they need to?
- Does time of day affect when they might be able to do something? If they can go to a supermarket, do they go at night/certain times of day as it is quieter?

- Could they go at rush hour? If not, why not? What do they think would happen if they did?
- Do they take another person with them to make certain activities possible? Whom do they take and why?
- What do they think this person can do?
- What do they think would happen without this person?
- Could they do the activity without them? Do they have other strategies they use to feel better such as carrying water when out, or the right change when catching the bus, listening to music through headphones, or chewing gum.
- Why do they do this particular thing?

Introducing the idea that such behaviours backfire

The practitioner can then move on to explaining how unhelpful behaviours backfire by discussing the following concepts.

- A 'vicious circle' develops.
- Leaving and avoiding can become part of the problem.
- Unhelpful behaviours are only a short-term solution for dealing with their problem: in the short term they feel better, but in the long term they feel worse.
- They will never find out that the worst feared consequence did not occur.
- ... or if it did they could manage this on their own.
- The less they do, the harder it is to do anything – and they slowly lose confidence.
- It is important to be able to face fears and overcome them – and rebuild confidence.
- The danger otherwise is an increasingly restricted life.

Vicious circles of reduced activity, avoidance and safety behaviours can be identified with this information and further enquiry related to the individual patient's presenting problem can be added as necessary.

The key thing to remember is the reason for gathering this information is to identify a target area for intervention in the altered behaviour area of the model.

Making links to treatment

Q

- What are their reasons for seeking help at this time?
- What are their expectations of treatment?
- If I could wave a magic wand, what would they like to be able to do/what would life be like?
- What aims or goals would they have for working on their problems?

The information gathered here gives useful information about the patient's reasons for seeking help and their expectations of what will be useful for them. Some people may be expecting a 'counselling'-type of approach or may have been told this by their referrer, and may not realise that there will be an expectation to carry out tasks between sessions.

✓ Practical hints and tips

Although a helpful and empowering process, any form of assessment can be an emotional experience for a person to go through, and can have a knock-on effect on a person's mood. The person ideally leaves the assessment with a sense of realistic hope and optimism that change is possible.

Choosing targets for change

The final aim of the Five Areas assessment is to choose a first area for change, i.e. one single area to work on over the next week. This first target should be jointly agreed, be relevant to the patient, and be likely to have a positive impact on how they feel over the next week.

The **Planner sheet** in Chapter 5 will help identify this useful first step and plan what changes to make so that it has a high likelihood of being an effective first step that makes a positive difference.

Other important aspects of the assessment

This chapter has emphasised the Five Areas assessment, and how it can be used to pick up patterns of symptoms that become the target for change.

Talking about times when the patient feels worse can help identify such patterns of unhelpful thinking and behaviour, and other important patterns that can help inform intervention. However, much more information is required to complete a full assessment. This will include how problems have developed, the past history, previous episodes and their treatment, key elements from the personal and family history, an assessment of mood and risk assessment and management as appropriate. Every assessment should cover a short screen for major psychiatric disorders such as psychosis, use of alcohol, drugs and smoking, presence of key people around the patient now and over the years – and more.

Key practice points

- The Five Areas assessment provides understanding of what is happening to the patient.
- It aids engagement.
- Crucially it helps the patient identify a first target for change.
- The Five Areas resources can help the practitioner complete a Five Areas self-assessment – but an important part of support is to help the patient identify patterns of thinking and behaviour (and more) that act to worsen how they feel.

Online resources

- LLTTF DVD Introduction: **www/livinglifetothefull.com** or **www.llttf.com** (free registration required).
- Planner and Review sheets: **www.fiveareas.com**.
- Five Areas assessment sheet: **www.fiveareas.com**.
- **www.llttfi.com** (service/practitioner licence required).

Further reading

Williams C, Garland A. (2002) Identifying and challenging unhelpful thinking. *Advances in Psychiatric Treatment* **8**: 377–86.

Williams C. (2007) *Why do I feel so bad?* Glasgow: Five Areas.

Chapter 5

Setting goals and monitoring progress using the Plan, Do, Review model

What you will learn

In this chapter you will learn about:

- Common problems when providing support for people using guided CBT (CBT self-help).
- Ways to help motivate the person and keep them feeling motivated.
- Choosing targets that are collaboratively agreed.
- Making clear and structured plans using a Planner sheet.
- Checking progress on a regular basis using a Review sheet.
- Using a Plan, Do, Review approach to help the person take small but steady steps forwards.
- Creating your own Five Areas toolkit.

Related chapters are Chapters 3 and 4, which deal with assessment and engagement, and Chapters 8 and 9, which deal with working with the various Five Areas resources.

Introduction

It can be hard for people to make changes to how they feel. Chapters 3 and 4 explained how the initial assessment can itself act as an intervention. Helping the person know why they are feeling so bad is the first step to helping them feel better again. This is important because it is easy for people with low mood and anxiety to be knocked off course by various set-backs. This chapter discusses ways of helping patients stay motivated and keep using guided CBT (CBT self-help) in spite of any problems or difficulties along the way.

Key Point

We know that the more support sessions a patient attends, the better is the outcome. Therefore try to help the patient stay engaged and apply what is learned.

This chapter also describes an effective model of working that can be used to support any Five Areas resource (or indeed any other self-help system).

Note: Because of the wide range of Five Areas resources, we have opted to illustrate the approach using the Big and Little CBT Books. The same Plan, Do and Review model can be used to support the DVD and the various online packages.

Starting out and *Write all over your bathroom mirror*

All the Big CBT Books commence with a *Starting out …* workbook. This introduces the Five Areas model and the CBT approach, and offers practical advice about how the patient can set up a system to use the workbooks effectively.

In the Little CBT Books series, the equivalent book is called *Write all over your bathroom mirror* and contains 15 practical things patients can do to get the most out of the approach. The 15 things are:

1) Set aside a time and place to work on your project every day.
2) Don't drink alcohol or nibble while working on your plan. Tea, coffee or juice are OK though.
3) Get energised before sitting down to work. Anything that uses your muscles for a couple of minutes is OK.
4) Read your little book over and over till you know it by heart. Write in the margin. Think about what it's saying.
5) Make a plan and write it down, step by step. Be sure to make them small, simple steps that you will be able to do.
6) Think about eating an elephant. You can do it if you take lots of little mouthfuls.
7) You WILL get stuck from time to time, so work out what to do about it in advance.
8) Your plan is like a new year resolution so don't let it fade away. Check your progress every week.
9) Get a lot of help. The more people know about your plan, the more help you'll get and the more likely you are to succeed.
10) Write yourself a letter from 10 years in the future – 'Thanks for being strong all those years ago'.
11) Pepper your fridge with post-its. Write I CAN DO IT on the mirror.
12) Imagine you are your own best friend and give yourself some good advice.
13) Think like an athlete and get coaching and support from anywhere and everywhere you can.
14) Plan your support sessions in advance – know what you want to say or write to a friend, a group, a counsellor or a doctor.
15) Write an agenda and use it in support sessions.

(Reproduced with permission from Williams C. (2008) *Write all over your bathroom mirror*, bookmark. Five Areas, Glasgow.)

Key Point

A free colour bookmark summarising these key points can be downloaded from **www.fiveareas.com**.

Factors that affect the outcome of guided CBT

Difficulties in using CBT self-help can be due to either *internal* or *external* causes. Internal problems are issues that are within the patient. External problems are the result of external circumstances affecting the patient or the reactions of other people. These factors are summarised in the Five Areas assessment shown in Figure 5.1.

Let us look at these factors in more detail.

Internal factors that affect use of guided CBT

Macleod *et al*. (2009) asked accredited CBT practitioners to identity factors that could predict how well or badly a patient did when using CBT self-help resources. The five key factors identified by more than 70 per cent of the respondents were all internal factors:

- Level of patient motivation.
- Feelings of self-efficacy.
- Level of hopelessness.
- High credibility/belief that the materials could help.

These first four factors can be seen as contributing towards the fifth factor:

- Adherence to and use of the approach.

Importantly, none of the first four factors is both constant and unchangeable. This has implications when introducing and supporting self-help CBT: that is, practitioners need to work not only to maximise motivation and hope, but also to enhance the credibility of the intervention and support offered.

Practitioners can also work in ways that enhance a sense of self-efficacy by helping people recognise that what they do can make a difference.

Key Point

The most critical times in engaging people are at the initial assessment and while working with them to ensure they come back for the second appointment/contact.

Patients therefore have to feel change is happening or at least may be possible. If not, then why would they bother coming back?

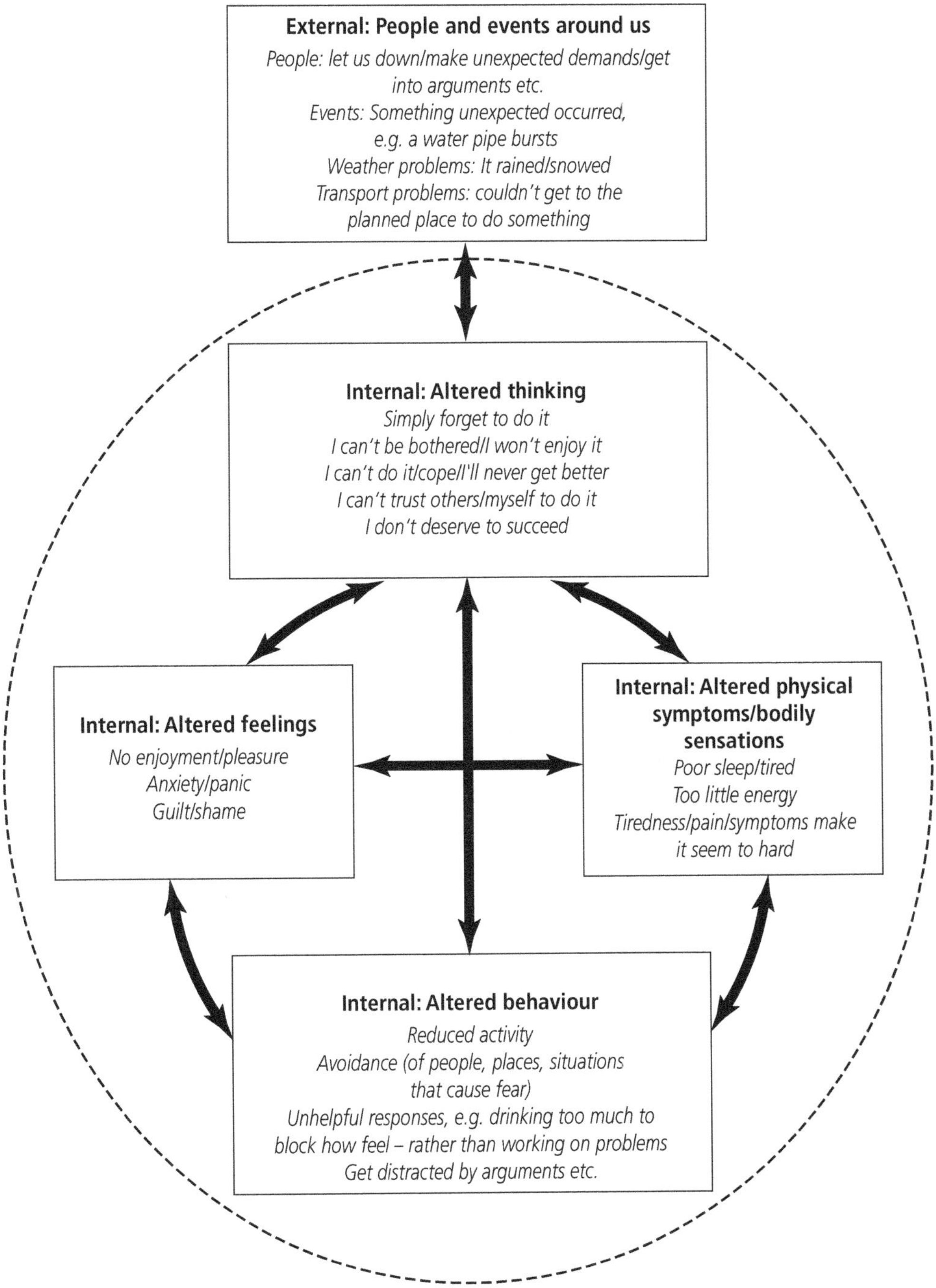

Figure 5.1 A Five Areas assessment of the internal and external factors that result in non-use of the planned self-help resource.

Boosting motivation

Depression reduces motivation. Anxiety worsens things by fostering avoidance so that it can often feel safer to do nothing than to take steps to rebuild confidence. The same problems are often seen in eating disorders and a wide range of other mental and physical health conditions. The practitioner can help foster hope and boost motivation in several ways.

Using the right tone to support

- Use your supportive relationship to encourage hope: show consistency, calm and realistic optimism.
- Emphasise your experience and credibility: show that you know how hard things can be, but there are things that can be done to help – even if only a bit to start with.
- Encourage the patient: offer praise when things go well ('Well done – it's great you managed to do that') and also when there isn't such a positive response ('I can see how hard you worked on things this week – well done!').
- Provide reassurance that you are there to help: People will sometimes do things because they don't want to let others down or because they like you. This may be helpful but practitioners still need to provide clear information that they are there as a support anyway. The patient needs to know that (within the confines of the number of sessions available) the practitioner won't criticise them, make them feel let down or be otherwise upset if they feel stuck or don't try something that had been planned together ('I won't be upset – this isn't like school where you get marked or have to pass an exam; we're in this together to try to find something that helps').
- Establish rapport and trust: Sometimes people need active encouragement and pushing – and this is easier if there is an established trusting relationship ('I know this is really hard, and I hope you don't mind but as you know we only have three more sessions, and I'm really keen that you start to get more confident in getting to the shops by the end of this. Is that something you still want to work on?').

Choosing the right targets

Key Point

Always refer the choice of current and next targets back to their own Five Areas assessment so the patient can see why what they are doing is relevant to them. A key factor is to choose something the patient themselves wants to work on. The key factor is that the choice is collaborative and not imposed by the practitioner.

- Goals/targets should be realistic and achievable.
- To boost motivation, plan some early quick wins: choose something that the patient can do in the next few days that is likely to help. This includes using workbooks that help them tackle reduced activity (e.g. *I can't be bothered doing anything/Overcoming reduced activity and avoidance*) or improving sleep.
- The target must be realistic. For example, can it be achieved within the time frame or a week or so (i.e. before the next appointment)?

✓ Practical hints and tips

If a patient wishes to become more confident, this is too large a task for one week. However, using the *I'm not good enough* Little CBT Book and choosing to create and use the 'OK things list' in the book regularly that week would be realistic and achievable.

Use metaphors such as 'You wouldn't aim to run a marathon all at once' to encourage breaking targets down into smaller steps ('Small steady steps all add up' that 'will get you there in the end').

Communicating the idea of regular, small steps

Another key to success is to encourage the patient to try not to throw themselves into changing everything at once. Slow, steady steps (Figure 5.2) are more likely to result in improvement than a highly enthusiastic start and then running out of steam.

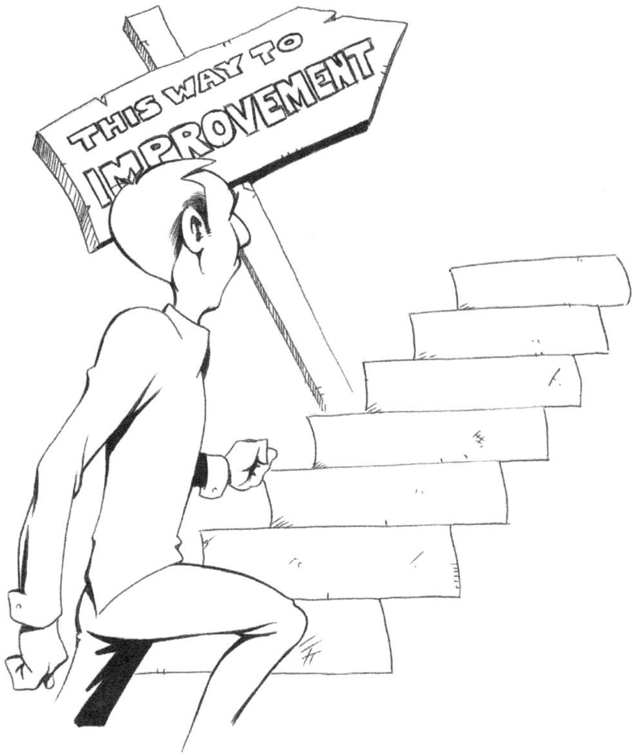

Figure 5.2 Slow steady steps all add up.

Unless the patient can create a clear plan and stick to it, change will be very difficult. Planning and selecting the first targets are a crucial part of successfully moving forwards. By choosing the areas to focus on to start with, this also means that the practitioner and the patient are jointly choosing at first not to focus on other areas.

Setting short-, medium- and longer-term targets

It is helpful to consider, explicitly discuss and set:

- Short-term targets: thinking about changes the patient can make today, tomorrow and next week.
- Medium-term targets: changes to be put in place over the next few weeks.
- Long-term targets: where they want to be in six months or a year. This may be well after discharge.

But what if the person wants to work on something the practitioner wouldn't have suggested?

As the Five Areas model is essentially a vicious circle, making changes in any area will help. A key feature of the Five Areas approach is therefore that as long as the target is identified as a problem, and is realistic and achievable, it is a reasonable thing to work on.

At the start of therapy, it's better to engage the patient in working on a problem they want to work on, rather than losing them by trying to encourage them to deal with something else.

Other interventions that aid motivation

- Help the patient recognise that low motivation is part of depression/anxiety, etc. Understanding this can help them see the undermining thoughts and apathy as an adversary ('Let's think what could really teach that bad thought a lesson or two').
- Use examples of others who have improved (while maintaining confidentiality). For example: 'I remember working with someone else who said the exact same thing. They found it hard to get started but when they did it really helped.' The key here is sensitivity – some people can misinterpret this positive statement as more evidence that others can do it while they constantly fail – so check regularly how people feel they are doing/getting on.
- Encourage honesty: 'Can we agree right from the start that we'll be straight and honest about how things are?'
- Use experiments: 'Can we try this as an experiment? Could you agree to try it for say the next three days – even if it's just to humour me – and then see if it has any impact? You may be right and it won't make any difference, but we won't know for sure unless you give it a go.'
- Get others on board: encourage the patient to tell others when they plan to do something. People will often do things just in case they are asked how it went.

What to do when people are too scared to change or don't admit the need for change

Some people have been avoiding things for months – sometimes years. They are scared stiff of change. An effective strategy here is to play devil's advocate. Agree that one option is to leave things as they are – but do say 'Before we do that, let's look at the pluses and minuses of leaving things unchanged – exactly as they are now.'

Try to keep the discussion broad by systematically looking at the reasons for leaving things as they are now:

The patient's choices	Pluses	Minuses
Impact on me now: • Physically: on my body • Psychologically/emotionally: on my confidence/how I feel • Socially: on my relationships and how I live my life		
Impact on me in the future: • Physically: on my body • Psychologically/emotionally: on my confidence/how I feel • Socially: on my relationships and how I live my life		
Impact on others now		
Impact on others in the future		

Filling in the above table is especially helpful when someone denies there is a problem. For example, a person may feel better if they avoid things such as by leaving a shop or by drinking heavily. Going through the recurring times when this response has occurred and looking at the short- and longer-term impact of the response on the patient and others will accumulate credible evidence that they themselves have put forward that a problem is present.

Key Point

Don't be judgmental when it comes to targets. People have to be ready for change. If someone doesn't want to change something, that is their choice. It is not our responsibility to drag a person kicking and screaming into change. They must want to make changes for their own reasons.

So, if someone can't or won't engage on important problem areas, a choice has to be made with them about either:

- Discharge ('Maybe then now isn't the right time for you to work on this – but I'd be willing to see you again if things change').

- Or to choose a mutually agreed other target ('Let's agree then we won't work on that area, even though it seems important. Is there something else from your assessment you think it might help you to work on?).

Remember that for some people with long-term mental health problems, these patterns have been present for months or years. Total recovery may well not be a realistic target, and the practitioner may be instead looking at small nudges that will move things forward even just a bit.

Key Point

It's better to help a little than not at all.

External factors that affect use of guided CBT

When a person is feeling depressed, anxious or overwhelmed, it is easy for plans to get knocked off track. Problems may occur because of:

- Other people: others let the person down or make unexpected demands ('Would you mind looking after Lucy? I have to go to the dentist'). Another person may become ill, get drunk and arrested, lose their temper, shout at the children and make them cry, or make your patient cry, etc.
- Challenging circumstances/problems/events: for example, something unexpected occurs such as a water pipe bursting, or weather problems ('It rained heavily so I couldn't go out for the planned walk with Sue') or something else came from left field to thwart a plan, such as a rail strike, a punctured tyre, flat battery or other transport problems, which meant the person couldn't do what they had planned.

Thus life's problems can be so varied. How then can we equip the patient with skills to respond to them all?

Bringing this all together: the Plan, Do, Review approach

The Plan, Do, Review approach (Williams 2009a,b) provides the framework on which change can be planned. There are two sheets – the *Planner sheet* (Figure 5.3) and the *Review sheet* (Figure 5.4) – to help the practitioner and patient plan and then review the progress.

The Planner sheet is completed towards the end of each session and helps the practioner choose which one workbook/piece of work the patient will work through that week. (Note: the practitioner can also encourage the patient to use this sheet to help them plan any activities they will do this week as a result of what they learn.)

Planner sheet

For completion DURING the support session

My notes **Date**

Which workbook/module will I work on next?

Plan to take things forwards

1. **What** am I going to do?
2. **When** an I going to do it?
3. Is my planned task one that:

• Will be useful for understanding or changing how I am?	Yes	No
• Is a specific task so that I will know when I have done it?	Yes	No
• Is realistic: is it practical and achievable?	Yes	No

4. What problems/difficulties could arise, and how can I overcome this?

Figure 5.3 A Planner sheet (available in colour A4 from **www.fiveareas.com**).

Key Point

The amount of space to write in what they plan to do has been kept deliberately small. It is large enough to identify one workbook to read or one task to do and thus avoids the patient making imprecise targets or too many targets all at once.

Review sheet

For completion BEFORE the support session. For discussion dated:

What task (s) had you planned to do? Write it here:

Did you attempt the task? Yes No

If you ticked yes:

- What went well?

- What didn't go so well?

- What have you learned about from what happened?

- How are you going to apply what you have learned?

If you ticked no: What stopped you?

- My internal factors (e.g. forgot, not enough time, put it off, concerns I couldn't do it, I couldn't see the point of it):

- External factors (events that happened, work/home issues, etc.).

- How could you have planned to tackle these blocks?

Figure 5.4 A Review sheet (available in colour A4 from **www.fiveareas.com**).

How to use the Planner sheet

- Post or give a pile of planner sheets to the patient.
- They can download and print off more free of charge from **www.fiveareas.com**.

- Encourage the patient to answer all the questions, and to carefully consider what might block their plan. This is one of the key elements of the planning process.

This same planning approach is used in the Easy 4 step plan (E4SP – Little CBT Books) and the 'Questions for effective change' approach (Big CBT Books). Both approaches help the patient draw up well planned and so-called SMART objectives (specific, measurable, attainable, relevant, time-bound; Doran *et al.*, 1981). This approach helps the patient predict what might prevent them from carrying out their plan and plan ways to react if things prove difficult. The Planner and Review sheets therefore reinforce this same underlying message that if the patient plans and reviews their plan in a systematic way, they will make far more effective changes than if they plan 'to give it a go this week'.

How to use the Review sheet

The patient is encouraged to complete the Review sheet just before their next support session. It then acts as their own agenda so the patient can make sure they get the most out of the support session.

✓ Practical hints and tips

If offering support by email or text messaging, ask the patient to email or post a copy of their responses to the Planner and Review sheets. If using email, practitioners can include the Planner and Review questions at the end of the email so they can be easily completed and sent back.

Adopting a problem solving stance

Regardless of the problems identified in the Review sheet, the patient and practitioner can work together to fix it using a problem solving approach. The stance taken is that it can sometimes feel very hard to change things. Every one can have all sorts of good intentions – but change will take time and there may be ups and downs. By using the Planner and Review sheets – and receiving helpful support and encouragement from the practitioner – the patient can stay on track. It also provides them with a structure to keep using well beyond discharge.

Frequently asked questions (FAQs) by practitioners on the issues discussed above and answers to these are summarised in Chapter 6 (see pages 106–107).

Producing your own Five Areas assessment toolkit

Quite often practitioners don't work in one location all the time, and may deliver assessments in a range of settings. If a practitioner wants to give a patient a particular sheet but has run out of them and there is no photocopier around, it can be frustrating as well as disruptive to the session. It can be helpful therefore for practitioners to make up assessment toolkits. This can contain blank copies of the Five Areas diagram, the various worksheets and copies of the vicious circles of reduced activity, unhelpful behaviour and avoidance (see Chapter 1 and all downloadable from free from **www.fiveareas.com**).

The toolkit should also contain the copies of the Big CBT Books or the Little CBT Books that the practitioner prefers to use and other resources such as the credit card summaries so they are all ready to hand out to patients. Laminated large copies of the diagrams and large print versions of any clinical measures or reading information are also helpful tools. Ensure that a copy of the scales used for scoring any measures is also available.

✓ Practical hints and tips

Write on the master copy of documents, resources and workbooks in yellow highlighter pen. This does not come through in photocopying, but stops the last copy being used without realising it's the last one. A laminated copy of these may also be kept as a back up.

Chapter 8 gives some more information on additional things to go in a practitioner's resource pack.

Key practice points

- It is hard for people to change when they experience low mood and anxiety – even more so when problems are long term.
- Helping people change requires a key plan. This involves the use of so-called SMART objectives.
- The Planner and Review sheets are an attractive way of operationalising and working to create so-called SMART objectives.
- The Plan, Do, Review model (Williams 2009a,b) can be used to plan any self-help approach, or any other activity.
- The patient themselves should lead this process – and can continue the approach well after discharge.

Next steps

- Read the practitioner FAQs at the end of this chapter, and add any additional common questions and answers.
- Complete the free online practitioner training modules at **www.llttf.com** or **www.fiveareastraining.com**.
- Sign up to the practitioner forum at **www.llttf.com** to swap experiences and ask questions.

References

Doran GT. (1981) There's a S.M.A.R.T. way to write management's goals and objectives. *Management Review* **70**(11).

Macleod M, Martinez R, Williams CJ. (2009) Cognitive behaviour therapy self-help: who does it help and what are its drawbacks? *Behavioural and Cognitive Psychotherapy* **37**: 61–72.

Williams CJ. (2009a) Planner sheet: download (free). Available at: **www.fiveareas.com**.

Williams CJ. (2009b) Review sheet: download (free). Available at: **www.fiveareas.com**.

Further reading

Macleod M, Martinez R, Williams CJ. (2009) Cognitive behaviour therapy self-help: who does it help and what are its drawbacks? *Behavioural and Cognitive Psychotherapy* **37**: 61–72.

Miller AF, Cunningham JA. (1981) How to avoid costly job mismatches. *Management Review* **70**(11).

Williams CJ. (2008) *Write all over your bathroom mirror and 14 other ways to get the most out of the little books*. Glasgow: Five Areas.

Chapter 6

Offering structured support face to face and by telephone or email

What you will learn

In this chapter you will learn about:

- The importance of providing structured support to people use guided CBT resources.
- Various ways of delivering that support.
- What to cover when offering support in 10, 30 and 60 minutes.
- Using protocolised scripts and checklists to ensure support is delivered in a consistent way.
- Preparing for discharge by helping the patient plan ongoing self-reviews.
- Helpful responses to common practitioner dilemmas.

Why support matters

It can be difficult for patients to use guided cognitive behavioural therapy (CBT). They may forget to use the resources or may be distracted by new crises or by the everyday demands of life, and struggle to set aside time to work on their difficulties. Symptoms of depression and anxiety make it seem hard to stay focused on being motivated to change. Support matters greatly in overcoming these challenges, and although some individuals can make very good use of CBT self-help resources by themselves, overall, the results using written CBT self-help for depression are far better and much more powerful when additional support is offered. The same may also be true of computer packages; however, increasingly these provide automated supports, forums and newsletters which also offer support.

The focus of this chapter is how to structure and deliver the support so that it is effective.

What is structured support?

The term 'support' can mean different things to different people. It includes general encouragement and reminders in case patients forget to use the self-help resources. However, crucially, for support to be effective, it needs to be **structured and planned**.

Key Point

Structured support provides a step-by-step approach, with ongoing identification of problems and active problem solving to overcome difficulties. The Plan, Do, Review model (Williams 2009a,b) provides a helpful means to deliver support in such a structured way and operationalises the so-called SMART objectives (see Chapter 5).

The Plan, Do, Review approach provides a systematic way of providing structured support. It utilises clear and specific targets, creates a step-by-step plan, anticipates problems and regularly reviews progress. The approach can be communicated using a variety of effective methods of support – each having its own advantages and disadvantages. But the central communications around that support are focused on using the Plan, Do, Review approach.

Support can be delivered as:

- Face to face support.
- Telephone support.
- Online/email delivered support.

Face to face support

The traditional way of delivering 'talking therapies' is via face to face meetings – where the practitioner and patient meet to work on problems.

Advantages of face to face support

- The face to face contact may add to the feeling of a personal connection and aid the development of a strong therapeutic relationship.
- The act of having to get ready and come to an appointment helps activate activity and 'get the person going' – and this is therapeutic in its own way.
- Because both the practitioner and patient are in the same room, assessment can helpfully examine body language, clothing/hygiene and the behaviour of the person (and anyone accompanying them).
- Practitioners, patients and often referrers are used to and are familiar with this way of working – and many patients have an expectation that this is how they will receive help.

Disadvantages of face to face support

- It can be scary for some people to attend an appointment, for example those with low mood and significant reduced activity and social withdrawal, and those with anxiety-related fears and phobias (obsessive-compulsive disorder (OCD), agoraphobia or social phobia) which may make travel or attending particularly hard. Similarly, travel may be an issue for those with physical/mobility problems such as pain.
- Money and the costs of transport may also make attendance difficult. A wealth of evidence shows the further away the appointment, the fewer the patients who attend.

✓ Practical tips to make face to face support work better

Make it easy to find the assessment clinic/location: e.g. provide a map, a list of local buses/train timetables and details of local parking, and enclose a photograph of the building where the patient has been invited to attend. This information can be included in a supplementary sheet to avoid over-loading the initial offer of appointment letter.

Make it easy to meet the practitioner: e.g. a phone call from the practitioner a few days before the appointment to introduce themselves. Alternatively, or in addition, include an information sheet about the practitioner that contains basic information such as the practitioner's name, and include a photograph and description of qualifications (to enhance credibility and establish relevant expertise).

Make the idea of having the assessment less scary: e.g. provide clear information of how long it will last, its purpose and duration.

Key Point

Making appointments seem less scary:

- Say 'You can bring a friend or relative along if you would like.'
- Say 'If you would find it difficult coming to see me, I can also offer the same assessment by phone if you prefer that. Tell me how I can best help.'

Some low intensity services try to balance the costs and benefits mentioned above by offering an initial face to face appointment to establish a relationship – and following this with telephone-based appointments. Similarly, many use a phased protocol where the initial couple of sessions are delivered face to face, followed by telephone support after that.

Telephone-based support

Telephone-based support is equally effective as face to face support as a way of offering both high intensity and guided CBT.

Advantages of telephone-based support

- It is possible to form a strong therapeutic relationship over the phone.
- Making a phone call at the time the patient wants provides added flexibility and may engage those who would otherwise struggle to attend face to face appointments.
- It is easier to keep the session to time than in face to face meetings.

- Telephone support is useful if the patient has work commitments or childcare considerations, or is a carer of another person, for example, which could make travel to regular clinic-based appointments difficult.
- The approach can be especially useful if the person is too scared, depressed or physically unwell to attend otherwise.
- Simple, low cost methods such as sending a text reminder the day before the call can also be used. The same approach can also be used for face to face meetings.

Disadvantages of telephone-based support

- Some people do not answer the phone if the incoming call shows up as 'Number withheld' – as often happens with health service phone lines. Warn them if this is the case.
- It may be harder to establish a relationship with the patient if you have never met (see hints below).
- The patient may forget they are expecting a call and not be in. This seems more common than would occur with a face to face appointment; therefore text reminders are very useful as a memory jogger.
- Distractions may more easily occur, making it hard to talk (e.g. if an unexpected visitor drops in, or a child or pet is suddenly sick).
- Speaking on the telephone may not offer much privacy if there are other people around. So, for example, others may overhear what is said when using a fixed telephone line in a lounge or hall. This may lead to embarrassment or avoidance of discussion of important topics.
- Children and others in the patient's care may distract them from the conversation (e.g. a toddler tugging on their leg or wanting to play).
- Money and cost may be an issue. So, for example, not everyone has a fixed line at home although most people in this situation possess a mobile phone. Even though the service should initiate the call, and therefore foot this cost, there are still service charges and line rental charges for the patient to consider.
- People can forget to give new mobile numbers to the service. Check contact details on a regular basis, e.g. at the start, mid-way and at the end of the intervention.

Note:

Text message reminders are a useful way of offering support but do not provide sufficient flexibility for the detailed planning required to help people follow the Plan, Do and Review approach by themselves.

✓ Practical tips to make telephone support work better

Provide an practitioner information sheet with a photo (as described above), and a brief description of the support worker, their experience and qualifications. This adds credibility and can help the person to get a sense of their support worker and build a relationship.

Consciously work on establishing a relationship on the phone. Verbal communication skills can be used to show empathy and understanding and ensure that the patient feels that the support worker is listening and interested in what they are saying.

Agree an 'escape phrase' that the patient can say if it is inconvenient for them to speak. For example they could choose to use a phrase such as 'It is cold this time of year isn't it?', which would lead the practitioner to understand that they will wait for the patient to contact again for the next appointment.

Agree what to say if someone else answers the phone, e.g. 'It's Jane here for the appointment' or, if the patient prefers anonymity, 'Sorry, I seem to have got the wrong person'.

Make the most of the phone appointment by sending a text reminder the day before and perhaps on the day of the appointment (if the person agrees). Services can reduce costs by buying blocks of text messages from telephone providers.

Help reduce costs by always phoning the person and initiating the call at a pre-agreed scheduled time. Be aware of added costs to them if they are overseas, e.g. on holiday.

Agree a back-up means of contacting the patient (e.g. by letter or email) if, for whatever reason, the phone number becomes inaccessible.

Online and email support

More and more people have internet access – on home computers, at work or via telephone, television or mobile devices. Approaches include:

- *Synchronous* approaches: where the support is given live and there are immediate responses to questions, etc. This includes live chat/instant messenger/videoconferencing services.
- *Asynchronous* approaches: where the support is sent out but may be read at a later time and when convenient to the patient, e.g. a bulletin/message board such as that used on **www.llttf.com/www.llttfi.com**, or email.

Advantages of online/email support

- The support contact can be immediate (live chat) and responsive – mimicking key aspects of a two-way 'live' conversation.

- Email may be less 'personal' and less immediately scary than telephone or face to face contact. Some people may prefer this added 'distance' as something they feel they can cope with.
- Email and bulletin boards (asynchronous approaches) can be dipped into when the patient is free – and means they can still engage in support even if they are busy during normal working hours.
- Bulletin boards provide access to additional real-life comments from fellow sufferers – supportive comments and advice – and provides useful vicarious learning as well as somewhere the patient can potentially ask questions themselves.
- Software such as Skype, which combines voice and videoconferencing at low/no cost, via a computer has the added advantage of being able to see the person as well as hearing them. This can be expected to enhance the therapeutic relationship.
- Computer-based packages (cCBT) seem likely to increasingly include the ability to automate support – so that responsive emails that specifically address the progress and needs of the patient are sent on a regular basis. These can also motivate and remind them to use the cCBT package or other resource.

Disadvantages of online/email support

- Live chat/instant messaging is not as spontaneous as live telephone conversation – and typing is not as fast a mode of communication for many people.
- Emails (especially automated emails) are prone to being allocated to junk mail folders and may lack the individual flexibility (and mis-spellings!) a human can provide.
- Many NHS IT policies specifically ban emails being sent to patients. These policies will undoubtedly be modified in the coming years as managers recognise the advantages of such contacts. Many workers may initially worry that email is not as safe as other methods, but logically, letters can also be read by others, or even be delivered to the wrong house, and there are ways of maximising the likelihood that emails arrive as intended.
- Many NHS IT systems block live video/sound being transmitted over their servers, thereby preventing contacts using videoconferencing facilities of services such as Skype. Some have rules that prevent Skype or similar software being loaded. If a practitioner faces this problem, it is worth discussing requirements with the local IT governance officers to try to obtain permission to get access using acceptable technologies (see also below).

To address current NHS IT rules and regulations:

- Inform and 'sell' the benefits of allowing approaches such as email and videoconferencing to IT departments.
- Consider delivering these services (with the IT department's permission) using non-NHS infrastructure, e.g. the unit can have its own WiFi system using a commercial ISP or purchase a mobile broadband 'dongle'.
- Adopt a well thought through policy for safe and appropriate email/e-support, such as that produced by the British Association for Counselling and Psychotherapy (**www.bacp.co.uk**). Others are also available so check with relevant professional organisations.

✓ Hints and tips to make online/email support work better

Set up specific email addresses to provide support with (e.g. supportworker2@yourclinicalbase.nhs.net). Practitioners should not use their own personal email or standard work email address. At present, many NHS email portals make this difficult. They should ensure that when they are on leave someone else, such as a supervisor, can access these emails if necessary or be very clear that emails will be unattended for a specified period.

Ask patients to add the support email address to their email 'safe/white list' to avoid the support emails being sent to a junk mail folder.

Preferably reply to the person's own email rather than typing their address in from scratch to avoid emails going astray.

Set up the mailing application/package to automatically not include the text from the previous email (e.g. in Outlook go to the Tools/Options/Preferences/Email options selections, and then the *When replying to a message* drop-down menu and alter the default setting to *Do not include original message*).

Consider using template emails that contain key standard information (how to get help, how to download more Practice and Review Planner sheets) – which can then be modified and made 'personal' for each patient depending on their individual needs and progress. Examples that can be downloaded and modified are available on the various Five Areas sites.

As with support for all guided CBT – aim to keep it focused on using the self-help resources, and do not use it for informal chat.

- Arrange a meeting with senior IT staff and identify the online cCBT packages that may be used. IT may say that the default position in the department is to block all audio and video such as the Flash movies widely used online. However, it can also (probably) either grant extra privileges for particular sites (by adding them to an approved list), or can purchase an additional server to run a mirror copy of the site free of the usual restrictions (i.e. with the requisite additional software such as Flash loaded). Practitioners should discuss these options with the IT staff, who will be aware of the issues involved. The key point that needs to be stressed to IT is that delivery of an evidence-based patient service through this approach is a recommended way of offering such services. It is possible for IT services to do this if they wish.

Who can provide the support?

Support in guided CBT can be offered by a practitioner who is qualified in CBT or mental health working as well as by practitioners who have received training in supporting and using the resources. The key is to have support that is:

- Structured and planned.
- Specific – so the patient knows *what* they want to work on and *when* they will do it.
- Is chosen (jointly) by and with the patient – so they want to work on it.
- Importantly, given by a person who is trusted and seen as a credible source of support.

Such workers can include:

- Psychological wellbeing practitioners and CBT self-help workers.
- Health workers and health trainers.
- Voluntary sector workers.
- Social care workers.
- Professionals allied to medicine, such as occupational therapists, speech therapists and physiotherapists.
- Teachers: interestingly, a large survey of young people identified the class teacher as the person they would most wish to receive support from when using self-help resources.
- Prison officers and other staff.

In addition, trusted friends and relatives can provide helpful support and encouragement.

Carer/friend/peer supports

Carers and friends can help with various aspects of the guided CBT approach. A specific workbook aimed at carers is included in several of the Five Areas books (e.g. *Overcoming depression and low mood*, 3rd edition, and *Overcoming teenage low mood and depression*). A specific online carer support package aims to help parents and other carers of those with anorexia (**www.overcominganorexiaonline.com**). The intention is to rapidly develop more such websites to offer a generic carer support resource online. Such support can either supplement the work done with a practitioner (e.g. to help encourage the patient to read, learn and apply what they are working on), or potentially can provide another way of accessing support for patients who do not choose to receive support from a health service or other worker. In addition, each of these resources helps identify unhelpful responses (wrapping the wellbeing in cotton wool, or trying to bully/force them to do things) and instead build more helpful supports.

Completing questionnaires when offering remote support

Key Point

It is time consuming to complete a questionnaire 'live' with the patient, whether face to face or over the phone. ('Next can you tell me how you have felt for each of the following 20 questions … was that less than half the day, more than half the day …'). A more time efficient solution needs to be found, and the solutions will vary with the type of support provided.

Some suggestions for completing questionnaires at a distance:

- **Face to face support**: It is quite common for patients to be asked to complete paper-based questionnaires in the waiting room, before the start of the support session. In some settings patients are offered the option of completing forms on a computer when they attend clinic, or before they first attend. Such approaches can significantly speed up the initial assessment approach. However, we do recommend that questionnaires are completed the first time with support available from the practitioner so they can familiarise themselves with what will be required of them.
- **Telephone support**: Envelopes containing key handouts and rating questionnaires can be sent in the post as part of a welcome pack. The patient can then be asked to complete these before the appointment (similar to what would be done while in a waiting room above). They can then have the forms available for when the support worker calls them. This allows a rapid and efficient reading out of their responses to the questions (e.g. a score of 3 for Q1, 2 for Q2).
- **E-support**: Editable versions of monitoring questionnaires can be emailed and either printed out and posted back or completed electronically and emailed back. Note, many licences for paid-for mood questionnaires prevent editable versions being used. An alternative is to provide a link to a secure online site where questionnaires can be answered. Licences can be obtained to put questionnaires online like this if they are password protected and not freely available on the internet. Currently such sites are usually found in research settings; however, within the Increasing Access to Psychological Therapies (IAPT) programme in England many services are using approaches such as the PC-MIS online evaluation/monitoring service (**www.pc-mis.co.uk**).
- Another option is to have large print versions of the measures available for use by patients with visual problems so the person can see the question they are being asked to complete clearly. Non-English language translations can be made available in each base or posted to the patient by the service.

Agreeing how to respond to missed appointments

There are two main ways of responding to missed appointments:

- **View it as the rightful choice of the person** – and wait for them to contact the service again. However, this approach overlooks the fact that depression and anxiety themselves make it easy for people to withdraw. A more assertive follow-up offers many advantages – as long as it is not seen as intrusive and unwelcome.
- **View missing appointments as inevitable** – missed appointments and non-adherence occurs in a wide range of physical and mental health conditions. It is well recognised in depression and anxiety with missed prescriptions of antidepressants, and missed appointments for high intensity interventions as well. Some services offer so-called *assertive outreach* – and actively follow up patients again and again if they fail to attend. This is most often seen in services supporting people with psychosis. It is also used in depression in some services – especially in the USA. Active follow-up is also recommended within IAPT services in England. The advantage of this is that many patients are pleased when services keep in contact with them. It also allows people to re-engage when they feel able to (e.g. they can drop back for a few weeks but still take things up again when they have weathered a particular crisis). The main disadvantage is that repeat contacts can annoy the patient if they do not wish to engage. It can also be

time consuming for the service. Keep a record of attempts to make contact with the patient, and discuss these with a supervisor if possible.

✓ Practical tips for providing appropriate levels of follow-up for missed appointments

One approach is to specify a set number of reminder contacts, e.g. two letters, a text and two phone calls to attempt to re-engage the patient if they miss an appointment.

A different approach uses the initial assessment interview to include a discussion of how actively the patient themselves would like to be followed up. For example, quite often patients forget to answer the phone, or sometimes want to slow down for a time and miss sessions: 'Knowing yourself as a person, what would you find most helpful? I could either leave it up to you to get back in touch if and when you want – or would you prefer me to phone you/email you for a number of weeks – not to hassle you – but just to give you the chance to get going again. What would work best for you?'

The issue of the time spent trying to contact the person can be addressed by either sending emails, or, if using the phone, using automated telephone diallers to phone the patient repeatedly until the phone is answered – whereupon the call is picked up by the support worker. This system is used in some locations in the USA but we are unaware of similar systems being used in the UK. However, it is our view that this would work best with the patient's consent in advance as in the point above.

What to cover when offering support in 10, 30 and 60 minutes

It is not possible to cover everything that can be covered in 60 minutes in just 30 minutes. Similarly an appointment time of 10 minutes allows still less to be focused on. This section therefore provides a model for delivery that retains at each level and is summarised in Figure 6.1.

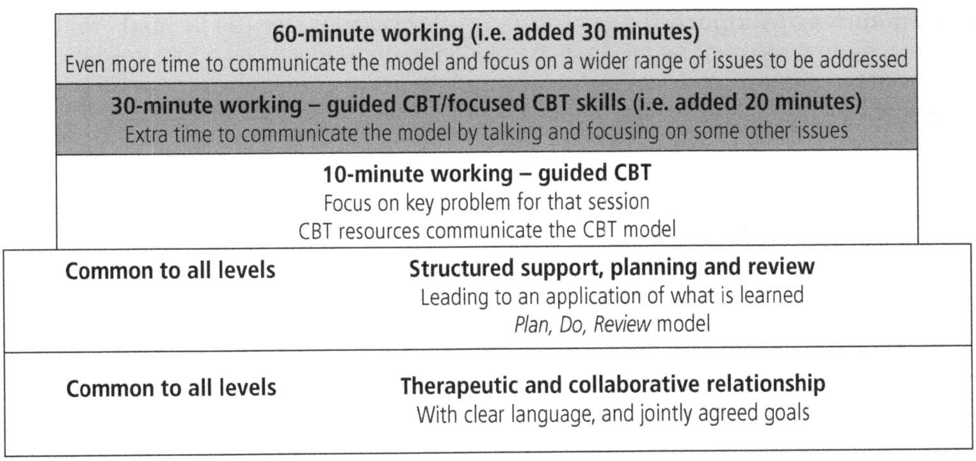

Figure 6.1 Relationship between high and low intensity CBT.

Key Point

The difference between high and low intensity working is that there is additional time available to communicate the CBT model and its application when there is 30 or 60 minutes available. Each level, however, requires establishing an effective therapeutic relationship, clearly communicated concepts, good communication, and a clear model to help the patient apply the Plan, Do and Review model.

Fidelity to the CBT model

Fidelity to the CBT model is achieved in different ways at different levels of CBT.

- **10 minutes of support:** The only way to achieve fidelity of delivery of the CBT model in this time span is to use structured CBT self-help resources which themselves adhere to the CBT model. The materials deliver the work and content of the therapy.
- **30 minutes of support:** Guided CBT (i.e. CBT self-help) – or the use of focused CBT interventions such as behavioural activation can be used.
- **60 minutes of support:** Here again, guided CBT or focused interventions such as behavioural activation can be used. However, expert-led CBT can also be offered. Here the fidelity to the model is achieved through delivery by trained and supervised staff working using a manualised approach (as recommended by the National Institute for Health and Clinical Excellence [NICE] 2009).

Structured support, planning and review

Underpinning any CBT work is having a clear structure:

- **10 minutes of support:** The focus should be on a problem identified in the patient's Five Areas assessment (by completing an assessment workbook/cCBT program) and using the Plan, Do, Review approach (see Chapter 5). The aim is to plan use of a single guided CBT resource (e.g. a workbook, booklet of cCBT package).
- **30 minutes of support:** As above – but using the additional time to focus on planning what to do and when – and then problem solving any difficulties.
- **60 minutes of support:** The same Plan, Do, Review approach can be used – with not much more time spent on this than in the 30 minute support. The additional time should be used to focus on working to a traditional structure of expert-led CBT – with sessions incorporating a formulation-driven approach, use of an agenda and homework, which covers much the same ground as above but in greater depth.

Therapeutic and collaborative relationship

This theme underpins work at all levels – however, the more time available, the more time there is for checking understanding, summarising and reviewing.

Key Point

The difference between high and low intensity working is that there is additional time available to communicate the CBT model and its application when there are 30 or 60 minutes available.

Using protocolised scripts and checklists to ensure support is delivered consistently

There are considerable advantages in using support scripts to help structure the delivery of the support. These provide a summary of key points to communicate during each support contact. Example scripts for telephone support, email support and face to face support are included in Part 6 of the book and are available for free at **www.fiveareas.com**.

Advantages of using support scripts

- Ensures that all key elements of how to introduce, support and review progress are covered.
- Allows consistency of delivery by a range of workers.
- Can be applied flexibly to avoid the discussion appearing pre-determined and stilted.
- Better outcomes are obtained by providing structured support than when just offering general encouragement.

Disadvantages of using support scripts

- Scripts can appear difficult to communicate if there is a perceived clash with the personal 'style' of the individual support worker.
- Practitioners may feel their ability to relate is reduced by the added structure required.
- Detailed scripts can be especially hard to use when meeting face to face. The danger is the support worker focuses on the ticklist/script rather than the patient – thereby not paying sufficient attention to the therapeutic relationship.

✓ Practical tips for using support scripts

Two types of support scripts may be used: very detailed ones where every word is scripted and read out loud ('Now, first I'd like to find out whether you've used any self-help resources before …') or a list of key points of topics to cover, which are then communicated by the support worker (e.g. introduction of self, what name they would like to be called, etc.). The advantage of the latter is the worker can use their own examples, phrases and experience as they cover the topic areas – while adhering to the structure to make sure all the key elements of how to introduce and support the person are covered.

Detailed examples of support topics for face to face and telephone-based support for the second approach are included in Part 6 of the book. These are also available in editable format from **www.fiveareas.com** so that teams can modify them for local use. We request that the original design credits should be kept on the final documents for copyright purposes.

Three key components to email and telephone support

Whether using scripts or not, in order to work effectively using email and telephone, make sure three key elements of the support conversation are in place:

1) **Offer structured support** using the Plan, Do, Review model described previously. The patient should be encouraged to write down their plan, and post, scan or email it to you to see.

2) **Keep the focus on the package.** This means referring questions and comments on progress constantly back to using/applying the various modules/resources and how these will be of help.

3) **Make it personal:**

- **Praise:** 'Let me encourage you …'

  It is easy for patients to become disheartened. Some of the types of things that can be said/emailed to help encourage a personal connection and support are:

  - 'Lot's of people think like that when they hit a first difficulty'
  - 'Hang in there'
  - 'Keep on going'
  - 'Keep working at it'
  - 'Step by step it all adds up'
  - 'Well done – I know it can be really hard getting started'

- **Always respond to key comments in emails**. When working by phone and also face to face as supporters we have 'real-time' opportunities to pick up on comments made by people, and respond to the concerns expressed. In emails, because of the tone/speed of the communication, it is possible to miss items that might have been very important to the person. So, the patient may have agonised over what they type for some time, and it's important to recognise this. In responding to email, telephone or face to face responses therefore pick out two to three achievements, difficulties or other important comments and mention them specifically. For example:

- 'It's interesting you mentioned that – that's covered in session x/that was covered earlier in session 1, so did you find it could be applied there?'
- 'Thanks for being so honest – I appreciate you telling me because it's important to know you're not sure whether this approach will work.'

- **Offer hopeful support/commiseration during tricky times.** Offering encouragement and acknowledging how things can seem slow/hard/distressing can really help. For example:
    - 'It sounds that things have been really difficult'
    - 'Even if parts of this aren't that helpful – hopefully some bits will really help'
- **Avoid self-disclosure of personal things.** Support workers vary in how they like to provide support. In general, however, we recommend that part of low intensity and high intensity working is to engage and support, and at the same time foster independence and self-confidence in applying the approach. In other words, practitioners need to avoid responses that can create dependency or develop. So, a neutral comment that can establish non-dependency creating chat might be 'The weather here has been awful also'. This sort of disclosure is fine because it offers something small about the supporter's life experience. In contrast comments such as 'I also feel depressed/was feeling like that when I had panic attacks' are best steered clear of. It is quite okay for supporters of course to have experienced mental health difficulties; however, there are dangers of the therapeutic relationship boundaries being breached if the discussion of support becomes too 'personal'.

Preparing for discharge with ongoing self-reviews

In several of the Hodder Arnold Big CBT Books the final workbook is called *Planning for the future*. This helps the patient identify what they have learned – and also create a plan to keep putting what they have learned into practice. Central to this is the idea of a weekly or monthly review day – where the person can review their progress and make adjustments to their self-care – while calling on others if they feel they need extra help.

The key thing to focus on in setting this up is to encourage the patient to continue using the Planner and Review sheets (given in Chapter 5 and available from **www.fiveareas.com**) each week and to keep to the pattern of Plan, Do and Review. This provides a structure for relapse prevention and for early intervention in case of relapse. It is sometimes said that the last symptoms to go in an episode of depression or low mood are usually the first symptoms to occur when a person has a relapse. Therefore ask the patient to note down the symptoms they noticed first and discuss early warning signs they may be able to pick up on in the future.

Overcoming common problems faced by practitioners using the Five Areas resources

Q The patient wants to talk a lot about their week or a certain topic, e.g. a crisis.

While this might be a reasonable response for one session, if recurrent crises arise then it will knock the patient off track from dealing with other important topics. Try always to divert them back to how the resources may help.

Possible response

'Thank you for mentioning that – it sounds really difficult. I know that in just 30 minutes we're not going to be able to change things too much – but what I'd like to suggest is that we try to pick on just one aspect of what's happening – and look at ways of trying to change that. Do you remember how when we talked last time we found that making small changes can all add up? Let's try and find one small bit that will make a difference now. From what you've said, this might include trying to use problem solving to fix the leaky roof, looking at ways of improving your sleep, and also ways of boosting your confidence. Which of these would you think might help you most just now?'

The Five Areas summary diagram can also be used as a way of structuring discussions when a patient is experiencing a crisis. This is a way of getting them to break down the problem they had at a specific time when they felt worse and works very well. The advantage of this is it allows the patient to continue learning and using the model even when things go wrong in their life.

Q The patient says: 'I can't be bothered.'

Possible response

'Of course you may feel at times you can't be bothered – that's a usual part of low mood. I can't guarantee results – but I do know that lots of people have been helped by this same kind of approach. At worst we hope you will at the very least discover some useful information about low mood. However, we hope that you will learn some useful and practical life skills you can use to turn things around in your life. Why not give it a go for a few weeks and see how you get on?'

Q The patient says: 'I've got so many problems – I don't know where to start.'

Possible response

'Sometimes it can feel like we're facing a mountain of problems or that we have a long way to go. The first thing to do is to get going – to take the first step. By breaking things down into small chunks you can move forward a lot. I'm here to help encourage you. You may have heard the proverb – a journey of a thousand miles starts with the first step. Well that's what we are aiming to do together – to help you turn the corner and feel like things are moving in the right direction again. We are actively choosing to focus on just one problem at a time to get the best results, and each area will have a knock on improvement on the other areas.'

Q The patient says: 'I've no time or I'm too busy.'

Possible response

'Sometimes we feel overwhelmed by demands of things we must/should or ought to do. We rush around working all the time with no time for us. That's what I'm asking you to do – to slow down – and plan life differently. I know you've said you're worried that you may let others down if you plan to put fewer pressures on yourself. But if you don't – what are the consequences of burning out or crashing? You owe it to yourself and others who care about you and depend on you to look after yourself. Slowing down and taking out some time for you will help you and those you care about. Can I ask you what advice you'd give a friend who told you that they were so exhausted from doing, doing, doing, that they thought they were going to burn out? What would you say if they then said they couldn't stop anything at all?'

Q The patient says: 'I feel stuck and I'm struggling.'

Possible response

'Sometimes people find this approach isn't for them, or they feel worse, or other things are going on in their life that makes working in this way not enough or right at this time. If so please tell me and also your own doctor if you feel able. But, the first step is to give this approach a chance and see if it can help. If you decide it isn't for you after that, then I encourage you to discuss with your GP what other options may be needed to help. For example, some people find that antidepressant medication can help them in how they feel – and help them get started in making changes.'

Q The patient says: 'I feel far worse and am suicidal.'

Possible response

'This approach can be very effective for helping people with low or moderately severe levels of depression. If you feel far worse than this, however, using the self-help workbooks alone won't be enough. Please as an urgent priority see your own doctor or attend accident and emergency. If you are starting to feel like this also tell us. We will check with you at each contact how you are doing using a mood rating scale and will also always ask you if you feel suicidal at all. We ask this of everyone because it's important we can point people to the right types of support they need'.

Task

As a practitioner, please write down your own responses to other frequently occurring situations that you have encountered here and include them for discussion in your own practice review.

Key practice points

- Both longer (high intensity) and shorter guided CBT sessions (e.g. 10–30-minute sessions) have much in common.
- Both aim for an effective therapeutic relationship, good communication skills, a focus on making changes to a single target area at a time, and using a structured approach that can be summarised as a Plan – Do – Review plan.
- The main difference is in the amount of time available to consistently deliver the CBT model. In low intensity working either guided CBT resources (e.g. books or cCBT) are used, or a focused form of an intervention (such as behavioural activation) is taught.

References

National Institute for Health and Clinical Excellence. (2009) *Depression: Management of depression in primary and secondary care*. Clinical guideline 90. London: National Institute for Health and Clinical Excellence.

Williams CJ. (2009a) Planner sheet: download (free). Available at: **www.fiveareas.com**.

Williams CJ. (2009b) Review sheet: download (free). Available at: **www.fiveareas.com**.

Further reading

Chellinsgworth M, Richards D. (2010) Good practice guidance on the use of self-help materials within IAPT services. Available at **www.iapt.nhs.uk/wp-content/uploads/iapt-self-helf-good-practice-guide-final.pdf**.

Williams CJ. (2009a) Planner sheet: download (free). Available at: **www.fiveareas.com**.

Williams CJ. (2009b) Review sheet: download (free). Available at: **www.fiveareas.com**.

Online support resources

Available free at **www.fiveareas.com**:

- Planner sheet.
- Review sheet.
- Editable telephone and face to face structured support scripts.
- Email support information.

Chapter 7

Delivering support in the LLTTF and other classes

What you will learn

- The benefits of class-based approaches.
- Why location and language are important.
- An overview of the Living Life to the Full classes.
- Helping participants put what they learn into practice between sessions using the Plan, Do and Review model.
- Common problems and how to overcome them.
- Other types of Five Areas class (e.g. the LLTTF DVD and Big CBT Books).

Introduction

This chapter describes an effective model of working that can be used to support the Five Areas resources (or indeed any other self-help system) in a group or class setting. Because of the wide range of Five Areas resources, we have opted to illustrate the approach using the Living Life to the Full class which is specifically designed for class-based delivery. However, other Five Areas courses are available, addressing the *Overcoming depression and low mood/Overcoming anxiety, stress and panic* books and the *Living Life to the Full* DVD, all of which can be used in group settings.

Historical aspects of teaching in classes/groups

The earliest known 'self-help' book, entitled *Self-Help*, and written by Samuel Smiles back in 1859, had as its opening sentence: 'Heaven helps those who help themselves.' In community settings, groups set up and run by those with experience of a problem area have been immensely popular and well attended by the public. Alcoholics Anonymous, set up in 1935, is a good example, as is Recovery International, which was established in the USA by a psychiatrist in 1937 for those experiencing mental health problems. Recovery International uses an approach involving an independent lay group with a professional supervision structure to promote relapse prevention. One of the big attractions of such organisations is the support people receive from other people with similar difficulties. This includes the chance to form friendships, swap helpful hints and tips, and realise that they are not the only person who feels like this. Knowing that they are all in this together, and the camaraderie and potential friendships that can form, can be extremely helpful. This sense of belonging and social contact helps the person tackle a sense that they are trying to cope alone.

Within healthcare services, group-based treatments are widely used and have led to the development of their own strand of psychotherapy. Some services deliver their entire support via groups, whereas others use groups as the default first option of treatment. This approach has several potential benefits. Group-based sessions not only offer all the benefits of peer support described above, but also provide an efficient use of practitioner time. So with two practitioners spending 90 minutes each (total three hours of staff time per session), up to 12–24 people can potentially attend a small interactive group or up to 100+ can attend a large non-interactive class.

Over recent years a number of classes or groups based on cognitive behavioural therapy (CBT) approaches have been developed and delivered in healthcare settings A class-based approach should have many of the same principles that make individual CBT self-help effective – common factors (warmth, empathy, being listened to) and specific factors (such as working to a clear underlying CBT structure and having a clear plan to apply what is learned).

Key Point

A 'group' or 'class' is not a treatment by itself. The content of the class as described here is based around supporting individual use of an evidence-based 'self-help' package. This CBT self-help book or DVD acts as a 'course book' and is the focus of sessions and homework tasks, with the group or class being the *support* method that is used.

A note on terminology

Throughout the rest of this chapter we have opted to use the word class rather than group. The rationale for this is to try to avoid the use of a term (group) that often communicates to those running it, referrers and also attendees that this is a form of group psychotherapy. Instead a major part of the Five Areas ethos is to emphasise that these are *life skills classes* and to advertise them accordingly.

The Living Life to the Full class

The Living Life to the Full (LLTTF) class is a life skills course for low mood, anxiety and other common difficulties that is delivered in eight sessions over 12 hours. The course is entitled: '12 hours that can change your life'. It acts as a supported self-help class – and is focused on eight of the Little CBT Books. Each session focuses on the application of one of the Little Books.

The class is developed specifically with the class attendee in mind and in collaboration with the same designer and script editor who helped deliver the Little CBT Books. The slides present information using pictures and a minimal amount of text. Each session and themed worksheets are colour coded to link with the particular Little CBT Book. The package has the following key features:

- Ages: separate slide sets for young people, adults in general and older adults.
- Languages: English, Chinese.
- Who is it for: the flexible structure of the classes means they can engage and be relevant for a wide range of people: people wanting to develop new life skills, or people with low mood, anxiety, low confidence or those struggling to cope or who are off work or physically unwell.
- Mental health promotion/prevention resource: antenatal classes, attendance management, schools (PHSE [Personal Health and Social Education] teaching) and universities, use within occupational health and wider workforce skilling situations.

Reports by Age Concern and the Young Foundation with older adults, and also reviews of the class with adults and young people have shown a wide acceptability of this approach.

The course sessions are as follows:

1) Why do I feel so bad?

2) I can't be bothered doing anything.

3) Why does everything always go wrong?

4) I'm not good enough.

5) How to fix almost everything.

6) The things you do that mess you up.

7) Are you strong enough to keep your temper?

8) Ten things you can do to help you feel happier straight away.

Practical steps needed to get the classes up and running

Getting a licence

The LLTTF classes require an annual licence (Box 7.1), which is available from **www.fiveareas.com**. This is low cost and provides a way of making sure that the disk is updated to the current version of the resources at each renewal. Licence holders receive the course disk and start-up pack, which contains:

- Four A1 size laminated posters to accompany key sessions.
- An age-specific set of *life cards* for a task where these playing card style resources are dealt out to attendees and introduced as 'the cards that life deals you'. The linked task is to complete a Five Areas assessment of the particular life challenges on the card dealt to them (e.g. you lose your job).
- A set of the *7 thoughts strips* for the unlucky dip task during the 'Why does everything always go wrong?' (thinking) session. Here, people are asked to draw one of the unhelpful thinking styles – such as mind-reading – which is then discussed as a way of introducing that style of thinking.
- A copy of the LLTTF DVD – the introductory section of which is played during the 'Why do I feel so bad?' opening session.

The CD-Rom contains versions of the course materials for younger people, older adults and adults in general, with age-appropriate examples and resources.

Box 7.1 Key elements of the training licence

The class is produced as a resource to allow professional workers such as teachers, nurses, psychologists, social workers or staff and volunteers of a charity to deliver the training course.

- The licence is for use in a single, local clinical or social service unit/team, voluntary sector local group or single school based at or working from a specific address. Team members can run the course at any location where they work (e.g. outreach clinics, community venues).
- The licence does not allow widespread use across, for example, several clinical teams/sites or schools outside the usual clinical service of the team. In that circumstance each individual team/school requires a licence. A reduced fee option is available when purchasing multiple licences for larger services containing multiple sites/units/schools.
- The licence allows use of the resources to run free access local groups within health, social services or voluntary sector settings.
- The licence does not allow use of the course in commercial settings. For use in commercial settings, please contact admin@fiveareas.com to discuss this further.
- The licence provides permission to produce paper copies of the handouts/worksheets/wall charts, and also provide electronic copies of the Anxiety Control Training (ACT) MP3 files for use only by people attending the course and the course trainers.
- The CD may not be copied and none of the resources may be emailed or passed electronically in other ways to others – including course attendees. The sole exception is the ACT MP3 file, which can be copied freely for use by course attendees.
- The CD is copyrighted and remains the property of Five Areas Limited and must be returned when the licence ends (or alternatively the licence renewed for another year).

Contents of the resource disk

The disk contains:

- Session slides (PDF) – needs Adobe Acrobat Reader (available free from **http://get.adobe.com/uk/reader/**).
- Handouts and worksheets that may be printed for use by attendees.
- PDFs of the four A1 posters for the group if further copies are required.
- Editable advertising resources so that class dates/times can be added alongside your own logo or service name.

- Example scripts for the main course – providing an idea of what can be said at each slide.
- A 'Read this first' document in each folder of the disk, which guides the course trainer through how to use the resources.

Key Point

When printing out the various handouts for the sessions, please print them in colour. The 'Read this first' document also highlights the process of how to print the PDFs in landscape format (by selecting Print, and then ticking the Auto-rotate and Center boxes before clicking OK).

Introducing and supporting the LLTTF class

Some people love attending classes, but others don't. So, in community settings it is often easy to fill LLTTF classes simply by putting up advertisements for a class. However, in some NHS or social services settings, recruitment to classes may be slower – especially if there isn't a tradition of working in this way. Choice is important in how the patient wants to learn, and how they wish to be supported, but this should be an informed choice. This means that if a patient is offered face to face support individually or in a class-based setting, very often they will choose the individual support, even though they may benefit greatly from what a class based setting could offer them. For some, this tendency to avoidance is because of lack of knowledge, and for others because of anxiety ('It will be embarrassing, I won't have anything to say'). This is understandable and if the patient's mood is low, being around other people may be something that they don't feel up to at the moment. However, it may be something that they would start to enjoy if they can be encouraged to attend.

Use an accessible label to describe the class

How a class is advertised can make a difference. Many services find that when they try to recruit people to attend 'Depression classes' or 'Anxiety classes' suddenly it takes months to find just 10 people. The term 'life skills classes', the Living Life to the Full class name, and headline '12 hours that can change your life' have all proved successful in encouraging people to attend.

The following strategies can also make classes seem less scary:

- Think about the location: for example, it may be more acceptable for some to attend a class in a GP surgery or a hotel, rather than a mental health unit.
- Think about the time the course is delivered: is it convenient – or does it make it difficult for certain people to attend? For example, parents will find it difficult to attend a class that is scheduled at the end of the school day.
- Give people expectations of what the classes will be like: 'The session lasts 1.5 hours and covers lots of practical things that people really need to know in tackling stress and low mood'; 'You don't need to say anything out loud if you prefer not to'.

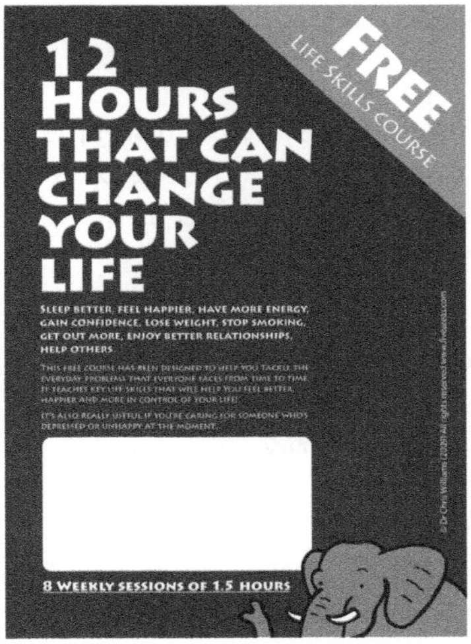
12 Hours that can change your life
FREE
Life Skills Course
Sleep better, feel happier, have more energy, gain confidence, lose weight, stop smoking, get out more, enjoy better relationships, help others
8 weekly sessions of 1.5 hours

Figure 7.1 Poster for the LLTTF courses and other classes. Copyright Chris Williams (2009).

- Start the session with tea, coffee and biscuits (the reverse of what happens in many classes): and also give people handouts/paperwork so if they prefer they can go and sit down, using the paperwork as an excuse for private reading towards the side of the room.
- Crucially, if the practitioner thinks the person would definitely benefit from attending a class, they should say so and explain why.
- Address misconceptions and concerns: if the patient feels anxious about attending a class-based setting, ask them what they think it will be like. Offer useful advice and practical suggestions.
- Provide different delivery styles to suit different people: for example, classes can be presented in a range of ways – some smaller and more interactive, others larger, less interactive and more anonymous (lecture theatre style, no questions to individuals, slightly dimmed lights etc.).

✓ Practical hints and tips

Keep some photographs of the room the class will be held in, and of how the room is set up. Obviously, you would need permission from attendees if they are shown in the photograph. This is a good way of selling the approach.

View a few slides from the content together.

Collect feedback from previous attendees and show these to the patient when offering support in classes. For example: 'I was really nervous about coming before I started the classes, but I have found it so useful and everyone was in the same situation.'

Making the class accessible and inclusive

Location

Location is important. The further people have to travel the more likely that attendance will be low as a result. Where the class is held may not be optional if the course trainer works in a healthcare service. It may be dictated by the rooms the service has available, or the trainer may be able to source a venue in the local community.

A proportion of people would rather not attend a building with an NHS label attached and prefer community-based options. The classes can be run from virtually anywhere. They have been running in colleges, in leisure centres, and in function rooms of local hotels and restaurants. Some locations can be very low cost (e.g. pubs and church halls). The key thing is to ensure that there are good local transport links and the venue is easily accessible for those who use the bus and also for those who drive.

Room layout: setting up a 'welcoming' room

How the room is set up can affect how accessible or daunting it seems. Some classes can run well in a hotel in a coffee lounge with settees etc. If using a more conventional room, try to have seats clustered in threes and fours around little tables to allow people to talk informally to each other if they wish.

Use the suggested scripts flexibly

Session scripts are included in the disk of the sorts of points to get across at each slide. This is not exhaustive – and is certainly not aimed at being read off directly (which would lack spontaneity and do nothing for establishing an effective relationship with attendees). Instead the scripts aim to give an idea of the right tone and content. It is important to have the session focused on the content of the books – and how to apply it (using the linked worksheets). Therefore having a structure and plan/objectives for each slide and the session as a whole is important. Although the scripts help the facilitator (course trainer) stay on track, the best way of using them is to understand the books and their purpose, read through the script, and then summarise the key points using the blank key points slides, which are stored in the same file folder on the CD as the scripts. Then, the facilitator should present the course flexibly in their words, with their own examples – and work with the comments and discussion from the class. Remember: this isn't a lecture so be prepared to respond to things that come up. In other words, the script is not slavishly followed, but the facilitator should aim to cover the key points seamlessly with their own examples and an interactive discussion with the attendees.

Using the posters

The four A1 sized posters are introduced in particular sessions and cover:

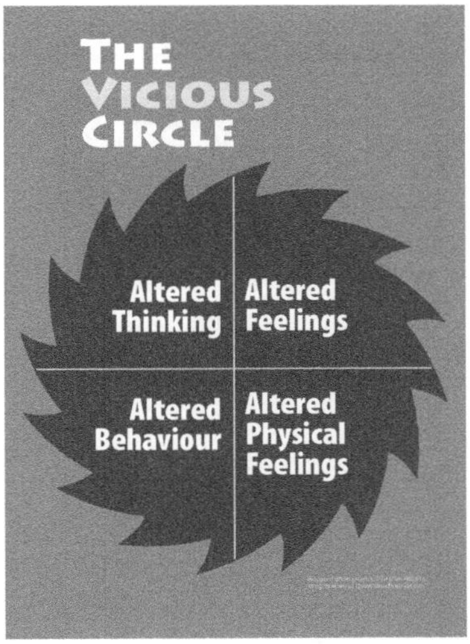

Figure 7.2 Poster 1: the five Areas vicious circle.

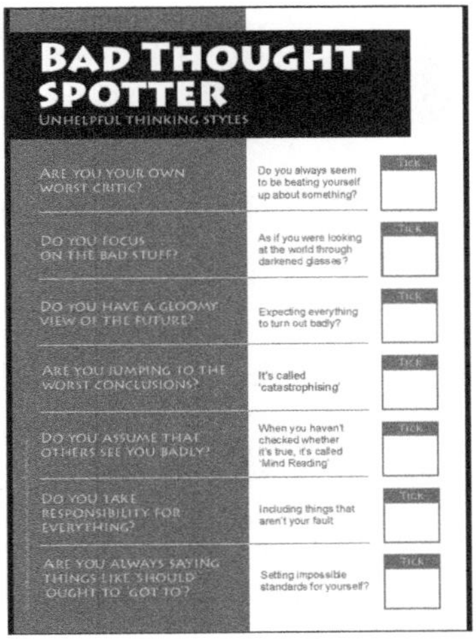

Figure 7.3 Poster 2: unhelpful thinking styles.

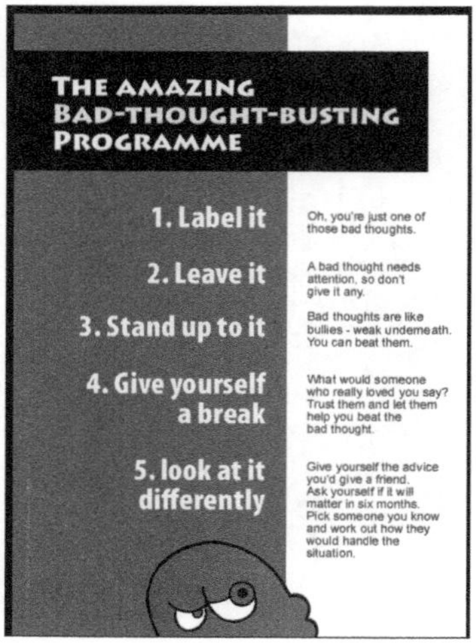

Figure 7.4 Poster 3: the Amazing Bad-Thought-Busting Programme.

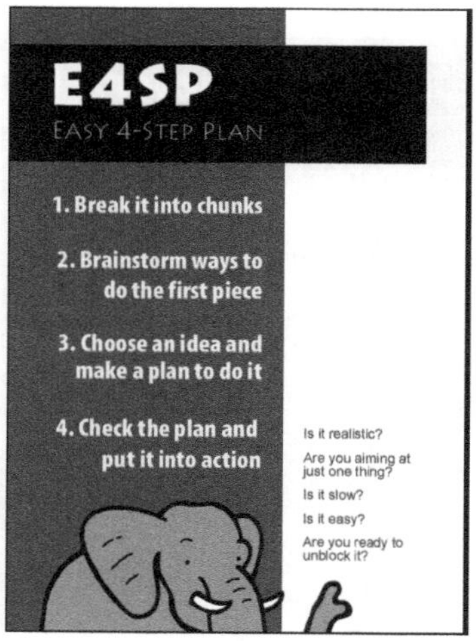

Figure 7.5 Poster 4: the Easy 4-Step Plan (E4SP).

In preparation for each session, the posters introduced in the previous sessions are put up on the walls – so that they can be constantly referred to during the session.

Using the colour worksheets

Linked colour worksheets are available as separate free downloads from **www.fiveareas.com**. They provide a structure to help the person practise and apply what they have learned again and again.

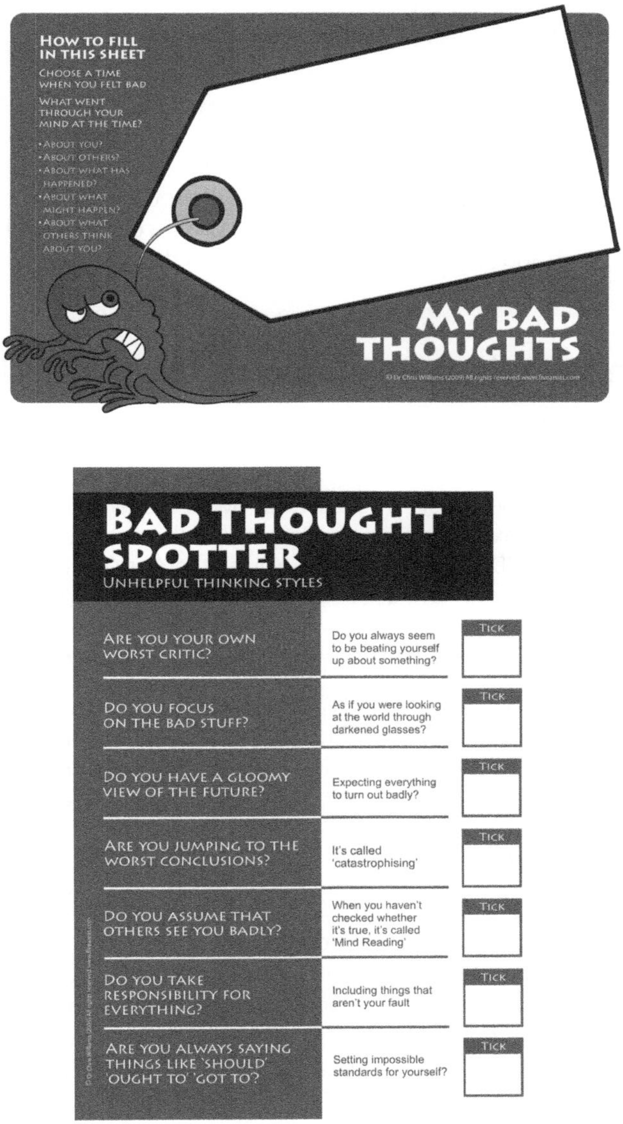
HOW TO FILL IN THIS SHEET
CHOOSE A TIME WHEN YOU FELT BAD
WHAT WENT THROUGH YOUR MIND AT THE TIME?
• ABOUT YOU?
• ABOUT OTHERS?
• ABOUT WHAT HAS HAPPENED?
• ABOUT WHAT MIGHT HAPPEN?
• ABOUT WHAT OTHERS THINK ABOUT YOU?
MY BAD THOUGHTS
BAD THOUGHT SPOTTER
UNHELPFUL THINKING STYLES
ARE YOU YOUR OWN WORST CRITIC?
Do you always seem to be beating yourself up about something?
TICK
DO YOU FOCUS ON THE BAD STUFF?
As if you were looking at the world through darkened glasses?
TICK
DO YOU HAVE A GLOOMY VIEW OF THE FUTURE?
Expecting everything to turn out badly?
TICK
ARE YOU JUMPING TO THE WORST CONCLUSIONS?
It's called 'catastrophising'
TICK
DO YOU ASSUME THAT OTHERS SEE YOU BADLY?
When you haven't checked whether it's true, it's called 'Mind Reading'
TICK
DO YOU TAKE RESPONSIBILITY FOR EVERYTHING?
Including things that aren't your fault
TICK
ARE YOU ALWAYS SAYING THINGS LIKE 'SHOULD' 'OUGHT TO' 'GOT TO'?
Setting impossible standards for yourself?
TICK

Figure 7.6 (a) Session 3: Bad Thought Bug worksheet; (b) Session 6: The things you do that mess you up worksheet.

The Worksheets can be printed off for free in English, Polish, Kurdish, Bengali, Chinese (simplified), Portuguese and Hindi at **www.fiveareasonline.com**.

Using the Little CBT Books

Each class is based around using and applying one of the Little CBT Books. It is therefore important that class attendees have access to copies of the books. They are referred to and read during each session, and tasks are completed that use the books (such as writing in responses to questions). These course books are also used to build on and revise key points between sessions. They are available at a significant discount for course licence holders.

A note of caution

If funding is limited it is possible to purchase a set of the resources for each person attending the session and collect them in at the end of each session. Please respect the copyright of the Little CBT Books. They are designed to be shiny and in colour to communicate a high quality product. Photocopying them will not do them justice and is likely to result in worse outcomes clinically. Photocopying also isn't any cheaper than purchasing the books at the usual bulk discount. Note that services can combine orders and request multiple delivery points to reduce costs further.

Practical delivery issues related to the LLTTF class

Welcomes, warm-ups and ice-breakers

You have probably taken part in some ice-breaker activity yourself when attending a training event or new job. How do these make you feel? Our own experience in this sort of situation is that we sit feeling slightly anxious as each person answers the warm-up question such as 'Tell us your name and the first CD you ever bought'. You sit there as slowly one by one people respond, and it is only when you have got this task over with that you start to relax and can listen to what others say. If this proves to be even slightly anxiety provoking for so many people, why should we ask this of people attending a class for anxiety and depression?

Instead, just have tea and coffee available as people arrive, so they can help themselves. This simple strategy does the work of settling in the attendees far more effectively. People begin to mix and interact in their own way, in their own time, and once the class has started to form, introductions can be made if necessary and will be far less intimidating.

Setting ground rules

Having ground rules can be helpful for everyone attending or facilitating the class, but rather than imposing a set of rules, these should be generated as an initial activity together. Covering things such as confidentiality and not discussing other people is important. Consider also how the people attending want to deal with people missing sessions. What ground rules are important to them? How can they ensure everyone can participate? How would it be if people are always late? How can the class avoid rudeness?

Doing this as a group task has many benefits, such as helping people attending to take active part, thus gaining responsibility and control. In introducing the classes (and selection criteria if being used), it can be helpful to make it explicit that you want people to make a commitment to attend every session.

How much self-disclosure is helpful?

One of the things that can sometimes disrupt classes is when one or more attendees comes in crisis and wants to discuss solutions to their particular problems. It is therefore important when setting the ground rules to emphasise that 'We aren't aiming to provide individual advice or "therapy" – instead as a whole class we will be covering a wide range of important life skills. In each session we need to therefore keep the focus on the topic being covered – so that by the end of the course we have covered everything. We therefore will need to keep bringing things back to what we are learning in that session. If you find there are really difficult things going on in your life can we point you to your GP or other support workers? And if people really find that things are proving tough for them – do chat to us before or between sessions so we can point you to other sources of support. This will make sure that you can get the added help if you need it.'

Two heads are better than one

Having two teachers who share the teaching can help (but isn't essential). It allows one to be observing, thinking and helpfully broadening discussion or clarifying if needed.

Key Point

The presenters don't need to be mental health qualified personnel. They do need to have skills as teachers, that is, being able to present, summarise – and facilitate a class. They also need to be knowledgeable about the aims, objectives and content being covered.

It isn't a lecture

The focus of the classes is the books, worksheets and discussion. The slides are simply there for reminders and emotions. Try to avoid always standing at the front as if this was a lecture with the teacher doing all the talking. Instead sit in with everyone else. Do get up from time to time, e.g. to point something out on a poster, but don't stand all the time. Remember people will only take away a few things from each session, so don't try to cover everything you know!

Don't cover up your own anxieties

Running classes or group-based treatments can even make facilitators nervous. They may try to cover this up by having too many slides so the attention is on the screen not the people, or by over-preparing in other ways. Watch out for apologising in advance (e.g. 'You might not find this applies to you') and for jumping in and answering questions if there is a slight gap before a response. Hold your nerve – and if the silence lasts a long time, re-phrase the question or break people up into groups of twos or threes to discuss possible answers.

What if someone becomes disruptive or too unwell?

Having a plan for how to respond to people who become too unwell or who are disruptive is important. Can members contact you between sessions, or only at scheduled contact times? Do they know whom to contact if they need help? Have they got the number for a local helpline or their GP for example? This information could be provided as an information sheet in the first session.

If someone is disruptive, how this will be managed should be something that can be discussed when setting the ground rules with the people attending. People may clash and not everyone may get on all the time. Ultimately, it may require someone to be asked not to attend.

Monitoring mood and learning outcomes

One of the folders on the LLTTF CD-Rom resources is called 'Session evaluation questionnaires'. These questionnaires include baseline and follow-up ratings, and end-of-session questions, to be used throughout the course. These resources provide useful feedback about how the class has been delivered – and the learning that has occurred. The feedback also allows facilitators to modify the pace and style of delivery.

In addition, some services routinely use outcome measures to monitor progress. So, in England in the Increasing Access to Psychological Therapies (IAPT) services, the *minimum dataset* of mood, anxiety and other ratings will be collected at every contact. In general, however, most classes run without using routine outcome measures. The downside of this is it gives a clear message that the class is addressing clinical problems such as anxiety and depression, rather than general life skills. To avoid implying this, some course trainers choose to re-label assessment questionnaires, so perhaps the PHQ9 and GAD7 might be combined together as a 'mood questionnaire' or 'personal health questionnaire' as is used in some services. (Please note the acknowledgements of the authors of the questionnaires must be respected and the content left unchanged, as required by the author's licence.) Other questionnaires may also be helpful that address a wider rage of problems, such as the General Health Questionnaire 12 (GHQ12, Goldberg *et al.*, 1997) and this also avoids the situation of potentially labelling the classes as just being about depression or anxiety.

Making sure everyone gets support

It can be difficult when facilitating class-based support to ensure that everyone attending understands the key skills being taught – and also that they are benefiting. If the classes are delivered as part of a clinical service then routine measures can detect lack of progress or deterioration. This allows facilitators to scan the scores for each person during the session, and look for signs of deterioration or increased risk. Facilitators spending time in discussion with class members and small group work is also helpful to keep an eye on how people are progressing (or not).

Scheduling a short telephone contact midway through the group allows for individualised chat and is used in some services. This can also be facilitated within the session time by facilitators going through the Plan, Do and Review sheets and having a discussion about how things are going.

Working on problems between sessions: Go for It!

Each class has a slide towards the end stating 'Go for It!' These three simple words represent quite a focus for the class (5–10 minutes). Here, attendees can come up with their own plan of how they will apply one thing they have learned that week. It might be to read the book, try out the E4SP, etc. The colour Planner and Review sheets can be used at this stage to help plan what they do, with the Review sheet being used for their own self-review during the week.

Different members of the class may be (and should) be working on their own different problem areas highlighted in their personal Five Areas assessment, and so may be doing different activities between sessions. Towards the end of each group session, when the main content has been covered, the colour Planner sheet can be used for smaller group tasks where people in twos or threes are asked to discuss their own plan for what they intend to do and when they are going to do it, with the other members of the small group giving encouragement and support.

How to use the Review sheets

Different services use the Review sheets in different ways. Most services encourage the person to do a self-review that week – and opt not to have a review time at the start of the next class. This means that tales of successes and problems are not shared. The rationale for this is that any negativity may suck energy from the start of that next session.

However, discussing (briefly) progress, problems and solutions can be helpful – if it takes a problem solving stance. So the suggested scripts build in a short (note: short) review time at the start of the session. Here though, attendees are encouraged to have already completed the Review sheet before attending the class so as to make sure that the class gains momentum and the discussion can start immediately. Feedback is then gathered from the class facilitators walking around these smaller groups and asking questions such as:

- How did doing your plan to apply what you learned last week go?
- Is anyone really pleased with how something went and want to share it?
- Did anything get in your way?
- How might we overcome that problem if it happened again?
- What have we learned that has been helpful?

Key Point

Between sessions, tasks should build not only on the content of the class or session delivered, but also on the patient's own problem areas or targets for change highlighted in their Five Areas assessment. Different members therefore may be doing different things between classes.

Online versions of the LLTTF class

There is a second chance for those who miss a class to catch up because all of the classes are available free of charge at **www.llttf.com**. This acts as a useful resource:

- For those who miss a class.
- For those who want to revise it between classes.
- For those who want to review what they learned as part of their ongoing self-care plan in the future.
- For use in schools and elsewhere.
- As self-directed learning independent of attending a class.
- As a practitioner training/skills development tool – to be aware of the key points of how the classes can be run.

Using the LLTTF classes with young people

A set of the slides are included that are relevant to young people. In addition, as the Little CBT Books have been reprinted they have slowly been modified to reflect the needs of various readers. One or two of the books currently still have examples within them that are more relevant to older groups. These can be addressed in sessions by saying 'Some of the examples given may apply to you, or people you know now, but also some of these may be more applicable for older people. It's great though to see some examples of how the same tools can be used at any stage in life. For example …'. Text will continue to be modified based on feedback – so please contact admin@fiveareas.com with any suggested changes to the class or books.

A second way of delivering a class: the LLTTF DVD

A second way of running the classes is to run discussion groups based around the LLTTF DVD. The DVD is available to view free of charge online at **www.llttf.com** and can potentially be projected from a laptop 'live'. It contains a full CBT self-help course that can also be run in a group setting.

A professional presenter and real people (volunteers from Depression Alliance Scotland) provide an audiovisual overview of all the main interventions. The resources can be used in the class by playing through a session in full, and then:

- Replaying the content is sections, with discussion to emphasise key points.
- Helping people discuss what is covered in twos and then as a larger class.
- Practising skills using the same linked worksheets used in the LLTTF class (available free of charge from **www.fiveareas.com**).
- Reading through the same Little CBT Books that link to each topic area.

Key Point

When the DVD is used in a small discussion style setting, no slides are presented. Instead the discussion and practice is focused on the DVD, the booklets and the worksheets. This works especially well where you have access to a TV and DVD player but not a laptop or projector. As such, it suits smaller more informal discussion groups. A key essential is to always link what is covered to a clear implementation plan using the same Planner and Review sheets that help structure the use of all the Five Areas resources.

Classes based on the Big CBT Books

Classes based on the second edition of *Overcoming depression and low mood* continue to be available and are currently being updated to a version based on the third edition.

Contact admin@fiveareas.com for further information.

Key practice points

- There are benefits of using the term 'class' over 'group;.
- Classes can be offered in a range of community- as well as health service-based locations.
- Because the classes are labelled as life skills classes, they attract people who might not opt to attend a 'depression' class.
- The class itself provides support; however, the process of change is again brought to focus by the book-based content, use of Planner and Review sheets, and a step-by-step focus on change.
- Classes can build confidence and bring about lasting friendships that endure well beyond the end of the classes.

Online resources

www.llttf.com: For access to the entire classes online delivered by Chris Williams.

www.fiveareastraining.com: 'How to' workshops for practitioners. Cover how to deliver the Five Areas resources one to one and in classes.

www.fiveareas.com: For the LLTTF DVD.

References

Goldberg DP, Gater R, Sartorius N, Ustun TB *et al.* (1997) The validity of two versions of the GHQ in the WHO study of mental illness in general health care. *Psychological Medicine* **27**: 191–7.

Further reading

Chellingsworth M, Williams C, McCreath A, Tanto P, Thomlinson K. (2010) Using cognitive behavioural therapy-based self-help classes to deliver written materials in Health Service, further education and voluntary sector settings. In: Bennett-Levy J, Richards D, Farrand P, Christensen H *et al.* (eds). *Oxford Guide to Low Intensity CBT Interventions*. Oxford: Oxford University Press.

Goldberg DP, Gater R, Sartorius N, Ustun TB *et al.* (1997) The validity of two versions of the GHQ in the WHO study of mental illness in general health care. *Psychological Medicine* **27**: 191–7.

PART 3

Resources overview

Chapter 8

Five Areas written resources for low mood and stress

What you will learn

In this chapter you will learn about:

- The various Five Areas resources that address low mood, depression and anxiety disorders. These include various different sizes and shapes of material, such as the Big and Little CBT Books.
- Ways of delivering these resources that are helpful to you and your patients.
- Foreign language translations and approaches that maximise accessibility.

Other resources aimed at helping people experiencing stress and low mood are the Living Life to the Full class (Chapter 7) and various multimedia resources (Chapter 9).

The Five Areas written resources

At the present time, health services are increasingly exploring the use of new technology with computerised and multimedia-based treatments. As a result it is easy to forget that books and written resources – an older form of technology – offer an effective way of communicating key information and life skills, and are highly acceptable to patients. Written resources have been used for a long time, with the first known self-help book having been published in 1859. Bookshops and bestseller lists are full of self-help approaches of varying quality. The key thing about a written resource is that it should be based on a sound cognitive behavioural therapy (CBT) model and principles, have a clear structure, and be user-friendly.

Advantages of using books

- People like books and workbooks. They know what to expect and what to do. Interestingly, book-based options are usually chosen more frequently over computer-based ones when patients are given the choice.
- Self-help books offer remarkably good value compared with other treatment options, such as antidepressants.
- They are easy to navigate – so the user can literally feel how long a book or workbook is and flick through it thus getting an overview of what is there and the key elements that will be covered.

- Workbooks get people writing. Notes can be made, text underlined and highlighted – or crossed out when disagreed with. Sometimes people only work out what they think about something by writing it down, that is, writing things down helps people work out things – and seeing things in black and white can provide a useful record of progress that can help when a patient feels they aren't making progress.
- Books/self-help materials are a bit like a new CD: some people may pick it up and play it straight away all the way through. Others may prefer to skip to the song they really want to hear. People do the same with self-help materials: they often go to the section they feel would be most useful to them at that time – workbooks offer that flexibility. That is why the Five Areas approach and resources are designed as a modular course.

Key Point

Recent research comparing the effectiveness of computerised CBT (cCBT) and book-based treatments for depression has found equivalent results across a large number of studies. This has now been acknowledged in the National Institute for Health and Clinical Excellence (NICE) Clinical Guideline 90 depression review (CG90, NICE, 2009), which has made it clear that cCBT and book-based self-help are equally effective options for care. They are therefore both reasonable self-help options to offer – and choice should be based on patient preference, i.e. by asking 'How do you want to work?'

Disadvantages of using books

The main disadvantages of using paper-based resources are around patient preference and whether the person can easily use what is offered.

- **Preference**: Some people prefer to work using computers, or classes, or with the more traditional face to face ways of working. While motivation is something that can change when people understand more of the rationale for using written self-help resources, some patients will not ever want to work in this way – and that is reasonable (see next point). Other options should then be offered.
- **Accessibility**: Problems of poor reading ability/literacy are not uncommon (Martinez *et al.*, 2008). Many people have developed strategies to hide their reading problems.

✓Practical hints and tips

If someone struggles or is reluctant to complete questionnaires such as mood ratings, it may be that poor literacy is a problem.

Significant work has gone into providing the same Five Areas content in different sizes and shapes so that they are attractive and usable by a wide range of people. So, for example, the LLTTF DVD has been created especially so that those who may struggle to read can learn in a different way. People have different learning styles and ways in which they like to learn something new. Some people find reading about it very helpful, some like to get going and practise, some learn as they go along or by seeing examples of someone else doing it. The same is true of the ways in which people use CBT-based approaches.

Readability and usability

Readability and usability are affected by a number of factors. One of the strengths of the Five Areas range is that it provides a range of resources with different structures that are attractive to a wider range of people than resources that are only available in just one format. They can also be combined to build learning in several ways (e.g. books and DVD, or DVD and computer – so-called *blended learning*, see page 138). All the Five Areas resources are designed to be easily used:

- Sentences are short and the text has been broken down into manageable paragraphs and sections. This means that learning can be broken down into chunks, which can be worked on without being overwhelming.
- White space is used to avoid overwhelming the person with solid pages of text.
- Jargon is minimised so that words are used in their everyday, commonsense way.
- Tasks are broken down into small step-by-step approaches that can be applied.
- Worksheets and checklists help structure 'homework', i.e. putting what has been learned into practice.
- Case examples are provided – so there is a human face illustrating how people respond to low mood and stress.
- Encouraging language is used that acknowledges change can be hard.

This work on accessibility has led to the development of two very different ways of communicating the Five Areas model in book form.

Overview of the Big and Little CBT Books

The Five Areas CBT written resources are presented in two different ways, which are designed to attract different people. One book style produced in the same format as the current book provides more detailed information, with longer workbooks and more interactive tasks and case examples. These are termed the *Big CBT Books*. In contrast the *Little CBT Books* published by Five Areas aim to provide short, to-the-point advice that picks out key CBT principles which the person is encouraged to apply. The key difference is in length. The Big CBT Books include more information. The Little CBT Books try to 'sell' the idea of making very focused and specific changes that can add up to make a real difference.

Both book styles use the CBT model – and both have clearly linked worksheets that encourage the person to try out, apply and practise the approach. However, different people may benefit from each at different times. For example, even when a person who previously enjoyed reading long, lengthy tomes engages in these types of approaches they may, as a result of decreased concentration, motivation or a sense of helplessness, benefit from the Little CBT Books at first. It's always best to ask the patient which books they would prefer to use, rather than recommending one type over the other.

The Big CBT Books

These larger format books are produced by Hodder Arnold. They include:

- *Overcoming depression and low mood* (now in its third edition)
- *Overcoming anxiety, stress and panic* (now in its second edition)
- *Overcoming postnatal depression*
- *Overcoming teenage low mood and depression* books.

Three more books are due to come out during the period 2011–12. These black and white format books are designed to be easily photocopied and reproduced at low cost. They therefore include a photocopying licence allowing them to be copied by the owner for personal use, in clinical work and teaching.

Key Point

Perhaps the best way of thinking of these Big CBT Books is that they consist of multiple shorter workbooks – all put together in one larger book. In clinical use, it is rare that someone would be sent the entire book. Instead, the person is offered support in using only those selected workbooks that address their particular problems or key areas highlighted for change from the assessment process or the *Understanding why I feel as I do* workbook.

Model for working with the Big CBT Books

The person usually starts with two workbooks (i.e. *Starting out* and *Understanding why you feel as you do*). These workbooks aim to help them find out how to use the course and overcome blocks to motivation (*Starting out*...) and to discover more about the impact of depression, anxiety etc. on them, using the Five Areas approach (*Understanding*...).

These first workbooks help the patient to complete their own Five Areas assessment. Building on this, the patient then chooses one or two 'making changes/intervention' workbooks to use next. Any workbook could be chosen as the first target for change – as long as the patient wishes to work on it – and it makes sense based on the initial Five Areas assessment. So, for example, the person might often start on a workbook that addresses reduced activity or avoidance, or poor sleep, as these are often good first targets that lead to immediate benefits over a week or two.

Figure 8.1 summarises this model for overcoming depression and low mood.

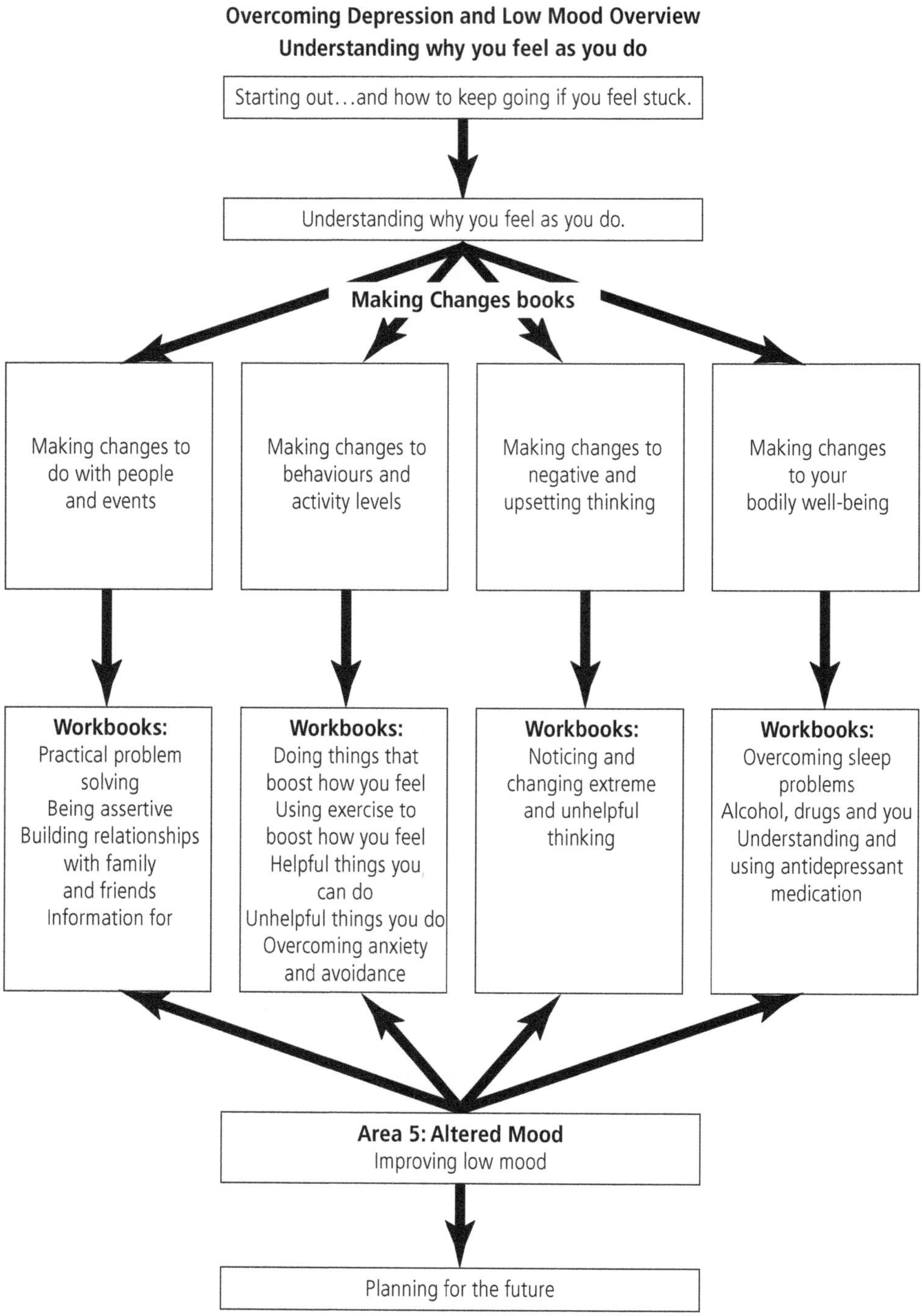

Figure 8.1 Overcoming depression and low mood: an overview.

Who are the Big CBT Books aimed at?

These books can be used with any patient regardless of age, who likes to get to the heart of things, and wants to find out a lot more about why they feel as they do. Practically, the patient must currently be able to read workbooks that may sometimes be 20–30 pages long, and they need to be motivated to record more detailed information in the diary-type worksheets.

Table 8.1 Overview of the Big CBT Book series

Big CBT Books – all come with a licence to allow photocopying	**Who is it for and what does it do?**	**Dedicated modules at www.llttf.com and worksheets at www.fiveareas.com**[*]	
CBT: A clinician's guide to using the Five Areas approach (C Williams and M Chellingsworth) ISBN: 9780340991299	Practitioners How to introduce and support the various Five Areas resources	Y	Y
Overcoming depression and low mood: a Five Areas approach, 3rd edition (C Williams) ISBN: 9780340905869	• Patients aged 15+ • Understanding depression • Tackling common depressive symptoms	Y	Y
Overcoming anxiety, stress and panic: a Five Areas approach, 2nd edition (C Williams) ISBN: 9780340986554	• Understanding anxiety/stress/generalised anxiety, and panic/phobias • Tackling common symptoms in anxiety including avoidance/fears/depersonalisation	Partial	Y
Overcoming postnatal depression (C Williams, R Cantwell, K Robertson) ISBN: 9780340972342	• Based on *Overcoming depression and low mood* • Case examples address postnatal depression • Written with experts in postnatal depression	N	Y
Overcoming teenage low mood and depression: a Five Areas approach (N Dummett and C Williams) ISBN 9780340946572	• Based on *Overcoming depression and low mood* • Case examples are of young people aged 12–19 years • Written with an expert in child and adolescent working • Emphasis on family/carer work	N	Y Pictures and handouts
Overcoming teenage anxiety, stress and panic: a Five Areas approach (C Williams and N Dummett) Due 2011[*]	• Based on *Overcoming anxiety, stress and panic* • Case examples relevant to young people aged 12–19 years	N	N

[*]Information as at July 2010.

Producing high-quality copies of the Big CBT Books

The Big CBT Books produced by Hodder Arnold can be photocopied for use in training and clinically. The following are important points to note:

- Copies made on local unit photocopiers are often expensive – and may be poorly presented (e.g. blurred, mis-aligned, and with staples that don't quite hold all the pages). Professional copying at a local photocopying shop is therefore preferred. Most shops should ask to see the licence allowing copying. This is given on the first five pages of each Hodder Arnold book.
- To get the best quality copies use one book: rip it apart and then guillotine the pages so you have a 'pristine' copy.
- To enhance the quality of the presentation of the photocopies, it is worth getting a quote from the copying shop for a front cover page for each workbook, e.g. use a see-through plastic sheet and spiral binding to allow easy reading.
- Large print runs offer significant savings. Quotes from formal printing works are often very much cheaper than photocopying shops. Services should consider combining orders to obtain the best rates.
- Each practitioner using the resources should have their own personal copy (not a shared copy) of the relevant Big CBT Book being copied.

✓ Practical hints and tips

If you are copying the new smaller-than-A4 format versions of these books yourself then use the magnify function the photocopier to increase the copy size to the A4 size usually outputted by photocopying machines (or ask the print shop to do this).

The Little CBT Books

The Little CBT Books (Living Life to the Full books) are produced by Five Areas. These are shorter, full-colour books, specifically designed to be colourful and 'shiny' and present a high quality and durable look. Because of this, photocopying is not allowed. Instead they have been costed so that when bought in bulk order quantities, they cost less than the price of photocopying the same sized booklet.

Who are the Little CBT Books aimed at?

Some practitioners seem to look at the little books and immediately label them as being aimed at younger people. In fact they are being used across the age range and a very positive report published by Age Concern groups, and also work by the Young Foundation, has commented on the attractiveness of these resources.

Thus people of any age can use them as, for example, mass circulation newspapers are read by 70-year-olds and also by those in their twenties. Its a question of whether the patient prefers to gain information in ways that get straight to the point, using material that clearly presents the key things they need to know, and that is easy to read and humorous at times.

Linked colour worksheets

Most of the Little CBT Books are linked to colour-coded (i.e. the same colour as the book) worksheets. These use the same attractive design as the booklets and are designed to provide the additional structure to encourage the reader to practise and keep practising the application of key CBT skills. It is also important to remember that each little book aims to deliver a lot of CBT principles – but does so with great clarity and humour.

Table 8.2 Overview of the Little CBT Book series

Little CBT Books – none comes with a licence for photocopying	Who is it for and what does it do?	Free linked worksheets at www.fiveareas.com
1. Practitioner resources		
How to use the Little CBT Books: a practitioner's guide (C Williams) ISBN: 9781906564100	Practitioner guide	1. Planner and Review sheets 2. How to use the Little CBT Book sheet
2. Patient resources		
Write all over your bathroom mirror: and 14 other ways to get the most out of your little book (C Williams) ISBN: 9781906564117	How to use the Little CBT Books	1. Bookmark with 15 hints and tips 2. Planner and Review sheets
Why do I feel so bad (C Williams) ISBN: 9781906564018	Understanding low mood	1. Five areas vicious circle 2. Five areas (table version)
I feel really bad! A guide for turning things around (C Williams) ISBN: 9781906564070	Prison version for understanding low mood	1. Five Areas vicious circle 2. Five Areas (table version)
I can't be bothered doing anything (C Williams) ISBN: 9781906564025	Reduced activity/ behavioural activation	No
How to fix almost everything (C Williams) ISBN: 9781906564032	Problem solving	Easy 4-step plan (two sides)
Why does everything always go wrong? (C Williams) ISBN: 9781906564001	Upsetting thinking	1. Bad thought spotter 2. Bad thought bug identifier 3. Amazing Bad Thought Busting programme (ABTBP two sides)
The things you do that mess you up (C Williams) ISBN: 9781906564049	Unhelpful behaviours	1. The things you do that mess you up target planner 2. The things you do that mess you up checklist (two sides) 3. The things you do blank help checklist (two sides)

→

Are you strong enough to keep your temper? (C Williams) ISBN: 9781906564063	Irritability/anger	1,2,3 Chill summary sheet
I'm not good enough: how to overcome low confidence (C Williams) ISBN: 9781906564–05–6	Low confidence/ self-esteem	What's in your head worksheet
I feel so bad I can't go on (C Williams) ISBN: 9781906564094	Suicide prevention book that aims to provide a more general overview of how to cope when the person feels things are just too much	No
The Worry Box: all you need to end anxiety (C Williams) ISBN: 9781906564155	Set of four books: • Worry/panic • Face it • Fix it • Forget it	1. Face it Planner sheet 2. Worry strips: included in the boxed set and online
Enjoy your baby (C Williams) ISBN: 9781906564896	Postnatal depression	Linked practitioner depression screening flashcards
Well-being		
10 things you can do to make you feel happier straight away (C Williams) ISBN: 9781906564087	• Well-being • Healthy living • Helpful activities • Behavioural activation	1. 10 things checklist 2. Happy Sheet Diary
Stop smoking in 5 minutes (C Williams) ISBN: 9781906564902	Smoking cessation	Support website: www.justfiveminutes.com
Live longer: have a heart attack (C Williams) ISBN: 9781906564–91–9	Weight loss/ management	
Reclaim your life (C Williams) ISBN: 9781906564889	Chronic physical health conditions	

Deciding what to offer – Big or Little?

It is important to complete a **learning and support** assessment – as well as a clinical assessment of the depression, anxiety etc. The key elements of this process are summarised in Box 8.1.

Box 8.1 Conducting a learning and support assessment

Key questions:

1. How do you like to learn/work?
   - Do you prefer short to-the-point information?
     (*Recommend the Little CBT Book course.*)
     or
   - Do you prefer lots of details and want to understand things fully?
     (*Recommend the Big CBT Book course.*)
2. Multimedia additional learning resources
   - Do you like to watch TV/video-style information?
   - Do you have access to a computer or DVD player?
     (*Recommend either DVD or online course to supplement Big/Little course books, or DVD alone if reading will be a problem.*)
3. **Support style:** How would you like me to support you? (*Describe telephone, email or whatever else is available in the service, e.g. face to face.*)
4. **Assertive follow-up:** Knowing what you are like as a person and how your low mood is affecting you, how much would you like me to chase you if you miss one or more appointments?

Flexible use – mixing and matching as required

The various resources can also be mixed and matched to meet the needs of the individual patient. So for example, a patient with low mood and panic might use workbooks from both *Overcoming depression and low mood* and also the *Overcoming anxiety, stress and panic*. Likewise, some Little CBT Books, such as those on low confidence (*I'm not good enough*) or anger/irritability (*Are you strong enough to keep your temper?*), can be used alongside Big CBT Book workbooks that don't address these topics. Similarly some of the Big CBT Book workbooks (e.g. on sleep or assertiveness) could be used alongside the Little CBT Books which at present don't address these topics.

Key Point

Ensure that what is offered is relevant to the patient, that they can use it, and that they want to work on the identified problem.

Sometimes services choose to work with just one of the Big or Little Book approaches so that they can get to know the resources well.

Telephone support: providing immediate access to book resources

Telephone support requires a different approach to face to face support. Chapter 6 summarises a strategy to introduce and support the Big or Little CBT Books resources by telephone. Detailed telephone support scripts are included in Part 6 of this book and are available free online at **www.fiveareas.com**.

In addition, when providing telephone support, an issue that constantly comes up is how to get the resources such as the Little or Big Books to the person in a timely way. For example, when a telephone support session identifies that the person wants to next work on problem solving, there is a delay of a few days before they can start as they need to wait for the workbook/book to arrive by post. This makes it harder for the person to visualise what the workbook will contain when the support worker talks through the content on the phone. Solutions to this problem include:

- Send out copies of all the workbooks/books at the start of therapy. The patient then can immediately pick out the one that is needed. The downside of this is that some won't be used (which is costly and inefficient) and there is a danger that the patient may get distracted and split their focus across many resources rather than focusing on applying just a few.
- A second approach that is more cost effective is to provide online access to the books. Both Hodder Arnold and Five Areas (see Box 8.2) provide licences to clinical teams that allow books to be hosted on password-protected servers. It allows the resources to be read immediately, and overcomes problems of delay. The downside of this approach is that it is restricted to those with computer access, or those who are prepared to visit libraries or healthcare centres where such resources are freely available.

Box 8.2 Further details for online access

- Little CBT Books: **www.fiveareasonline.com**; contact admin@fiveareas.com
- Big CBT Books: jenny.davis@hodder.co.uk

Linking the Big/Little CBT Books with other resources (blending learning)

People who are feeling anxious or depressed can find it difficult to remember things effectively. Therefore the support worker needs to use several different ways to enhance learning. Research into effective learning has shown again and again that learning is enhanced when it is active (i.e. when the person doesn't just read things – but interacts with it), and also when it is reinforced by learning using different modalities. The Living Life to the Full (LLFF) DVD and free online course (**www.llttf.com**) are both designed to supplement the use of the Big and Little CBT Books. Their content is described in more detail in Chapter 9. However, the key elements are:

- **LLTTF DVD**: modules on the Five Areas approach, problem solving, sleep and more. Real people who have recovered from depression (and who are members of the voluntary sector organisation Depression Alliance Scotland) talk about what they have learned using the Five Areas approach.
- **www.llttf.com** aims to supplement the various Big and Little CBT Books. It does this through a growing range of audio modules, and regular support emails, newsletters and forums.
- Additional linked **worksheets** for both the Little and Big Book series are available free of charge from **www.fiveareas.com**. These resources specifically allow the reader to practise and apply the key components covered in the books again and again.

Key Point

Whether using the Big or Little Books or DVD, there are benefits of using the linked worksheets. Many people also like to see how others face similar problems – and so benefit from the additional teaching modules and other online supports such as the LLTTF forum and newsletters.

Resource packs

Practitioners' Five Areas resource pack

Whether using the Big or Little CBT Books, it can be helpful for practitioners to make up their own self-help resource pack. This can be a folder or (preferably) a case holding file folders containing copies of the various workbooks, books and key linked handouts. This can then be taken to the clinic, on home visits, etc. so that resources are always easily to hand.

Practitioners working in a fixed centre (e.g. a day hospital, social services centre or telephone call centre) can store the resources in a filing cabinet. Any member of staff can then ensure the content is complete and updated at all times.

Patients' resource packs

Similarly, patients can be encouraged to create their own personal resource pack with completed worksheets, diary sheets, learning points, workbooks, printouts, etc. within a folder. The pack is useful both in the short term for organisation, and in the long term, as it brings together all the resources and things that have been learned for easy access if needed again in future.

✓ Practical hints and tips

Encourage the person to have one overview sheet of key learning points they learn throughout the clinical support. They should write down any new key learning points whenever they are recognised. This might be during a support session, when reading a book or when applying what is learned during the week.

Writing down key learning points helps them be retained and applied. It also provides a valuable summary for future use.

Keeping on track

An important aspect of the role of practitioners/support workers is to remind, encourage, help plan and motivate people to keep on track. Chapter 5 describes in more detail how to use the Plan, Do and Review approach to help people track their progress. A key element of this model is simply remembering to read and applying what is learned. Various practical things can help, such as encouraging patients to:

- Set alarms on watches and mobiles, use call backs from an alarm system on a phone, or set up reminder emails using the free Reminder system on **www.llttfi.com**.
- Ask friends and relatives to gently remind them to read the next book, go out, or complete whatever task helps them move forwards.

Notes for budget holders and commissioners

Both the Big and Little CBT Books are not subject to VAT.

Why buy in bulk?

The books can be obtained at significantly lower cost by purchasing in bulk.

- The Big CBT Books can be purchased direct from the publisher at significant discounts. To take advantage of this please contact: Jane MacRae, Sales Development Manager, Hodder Headline, 338 Euston Road, London NW1 3BH. Tel: +44 (0) 20 7873 6146. Fax: +44 (0) 20 7873 6220. Email: jane.macrae@hodder.co.uk.
- The Little CBT Books are very much cheaper to order in bulk than when photocopying. Services can combine orders and pay just the additional delivery costs to obtain greater discounted rates. Larger orders can also be stored in central supplies.

> Good practice example
>
> In Kirklees/Calderdale, the workbooks are ordered from central supplies in the same way as photocopying paper/envelopes.

- The Little CBT Books can be read online under licence at **www.fiveareasonline.com** by unlimited numbers of patients.

Foreign language translations

- **Little CBT Books**: Translations of the Little CBT Books are available in a growing range of languages including Kurdish, Chinese, Polish, Portuguese and Bengali.
- **Big CBT Books**: Polish and Dutch versions of *Overcoming depression and low mood* are available. Additional translations are underway. (For further information about translations please contact admin@fiveareas.ltd.uk.)

Increasing accessibility of the written materials

Versions of the Big Books and Little Books in a format usable by screen readers, and also large print versions, are available under licence from **www.fiveareasonline.com**.

Key practice points

- Accessibility is an importance concept in working with people.
- Resources have to be available in a format and delivery method that the person can actually use.
- Large print, non-English language and screen reader versions therefore complement the DVD, written and online courses.

Next steps

In order to use the books well, a practitioner needs to get to know them well, and should be able to give clear (and motivational) summaries of their content. It can be useful therefore to have prepared a summary sheet of the key features of the content of that resource. Table 8.3 is a completed example of a summary of the *Overcoming depression and low mood* workbooks. Read through this, and then complete the task that follows.

Table 8.3 Example: Key elements of the *Overcoming depression and low mood*, 3rd edition, workbooks

Resource	Summarising the resource for patients
Starting out...	'This workbook will explain how you can get the most from the course materials … and how to keep going if you feel stuck'
Understanding why I feel as I do	'This is the workbook to read first. If you can work out why you feel as you do, you can work out what areas to change'
Practical problem solving	'We often feel overwhelmed by problems/difficulties. You can tackle these one at a time using the effective step-by-step approach'
Being assertive	'Do you feel like you always end up saying yes when you mean no? This workbook will help you discover the rules of assertiveness and how to work these into your life'
Building relationships	'Those who are closest to us can affect us more than anyone. This workbook will help you discover how to build and re-build relationships'
Information for families and friends	'Would you like to ask a family member or a friend to support you? This resource is to give to that person, so they will understand more about how you feel and how they can best help you'
Noticing and changing extreme and unhelpful thinking	'When we feel down, we often struggle with negative and upsetting thoughts. Fortunately there are some good strategies to tackle these. You can find out more by reading this workbook. Lots of people have found this workbook helpful'
Overcoming reduced activity and avoidance	'When we feel low it's easy for us to reduce what we do. The trouble is doing less means we enjoy less and we can end up getting stuck in a cycle of reduced activity and reduced pleasure and sense of achievement. This workbook will show you how to tackle this'
Using exercise to boost how you feel	'Before antidepressants were introduced, doctors and patients often used exercise to give a boost if they were feeling low. This approach is now coming back as doctors have realised it is still very helpful. This workbook describes some slow steady ways of planning exercise'
Helpful and unhelpful things we can do	'This workbook will help you find out which activities help and which drag you down and keep your problems going'
Alcohol, drugs and you	'Drinking too much or using street drugs can worsen how we feel. This workbook will help you find out if you have a problem here and how to overcome it'
Overcoming sleep problems	'If we are not sleeping we can feel much worse. The clear strategies described here can help boost your sleep'
Understanding and using antidepressant medication	'Not everyone takes tablets for treating depression. This workbook will help you find out more about antidepressants, how they work and how they can have a useful part of play in your recovery'
Planning for the future	'Read this workbook before you complete the course to plan ways of putting what you've learned into practice'

Task

Now, as you read through the different books and workbooks, note down their key features in Tables 8.4–8.8 (Appendix 8.1, pages 143–147). From these, create your own two- to three-line 'motivating reasons' that highlight why it would be worthwhile for a patient to use each resource.

Use your summaries with patients to concisely 'sell' the relevance of a book/workbook and so that they can see how it would meet their own needs.

References

Martinez R, Whitfield G, Dafters R, Williams CJ. (2008) Can people read self-help manuals for depression? A challenge for the stepped care model and book prescription schemes. *Behavioural and Cognitive Psychotherapy* **36**: 89–97.

National Institute for Health and Clinical Excellence (NICE). (2009) *Depression: Management of depression in primary and secondary care*. Clinical guideline 90. London: National Institute for Health and Clinical Excellence.

Further reading

Gellatly J, Bower P, Hennessy S, Richards D, Gilbody S, Lovell K. (2007) What makes self-help interventions effective in the management of depressive symptoms? Meta-analysis and meta-regression. *Psychological Medicine* **37**: 1217–28.

MacLeod M, Martinez R, Williams C. (2009) Cognitive behaviour therapy self-help: who does it help and what are its drawbacks? *Behavioural and Cognitive Psychotherapy* **37**: 61–72.

Martinez R, Whitfield G, Dafters R, Williams CJ. (2008) Can people read self-help manuals for depression? A challenge for the stepped care model and book prescription schemes. *Behavioural and Cognitive Psychotherapy* **36**: 89–97.

National Institute for Health and Clinical Excellence (NICE). (2007) *Anxiety: Management of anxiety in adults in primary, secondary and community settings*. Clinical guideline 22. London: National Institute for Health and Clinical Excellence.

National Institute for Health and Clinical Excellence (NICE). (2009) *Depression: Management of depression in primary and secondary care*. Clinical guideline 90. London: National Institute for Health and Clinical Excellence.

Whitfield G, Williams C. (2001) Written and computer-based self-help treatments for depression. *British Medical Bulletin* **57**: 133–44.

Williams C, Martinez R. (2008) Increasing access to CBT: Stepped care and CBT self-help models in practice. *Behavioural and Cognitive Psychotherapy* **36**: 675–83.

Williams C, Morrison J, Wilson P *et al*. (2007) An evaluation of the effectiveness of structured cognitive behaviour therapy self-help materials delivered by a self-help support worker within primary care. Chief Scientist Office Study Report. CZH461.

Appendix 8.1

Table 8.4 Key features of each workbook in *Overcoming depression and low mood*, 3rd edition

Workbook	Key features of that workbook
Starting out	
Understanding why I feel as I do	
Practical problem solving	
Being assertive	
Building relationships	
Information for families and friends	
Noticing and changing extreme and unhelpful thinking	
Overcoming reduced activity and avoidance	
Using exercise to boost how you feel	
Helpful and unhelpful things we can do	
Alcohol, drugs and you	
Overcoming sleep problems	
Understanding and using antidepressant medication	
Planning for the future	
General comments about the book	

Table 8.5 Key features of each workbook in *Overcoming anxiety, stress and panic*, 2nd edition

Workbook	Key features of that workbook
Tackling your anxiety: starting out (... and how to keep going if you feel stuck)	
Understanding worry and stress	
Understanding panic and phobias	
How to start fixing problems and finding solutions (practical problem solving)	
How to ask for what you really need (being assertive)	
Learning to be calmer, less annoyed and less irritated	
How to get a good night's sleep: overcoming anxiety and sleep problems	
Using exercise to overcome stress	
Things you do that worsen your anxiety (unhelpful behaviours)	
Stress, alcohol and drugs	
Facing fears and overcoming avoidance	
Understanding and overcoming shyness and social phobia	
Noticing and changing anxious thinking	
Understanding and overcoming feelings of depersonalisation	
Overcoming anxious overbreathing (hyperventilation)	
General comments about the book	

Table 8.6 Key features of each workbook in *Overcoming postnatal depression*

Workbook	Key features of that workbook
Starting out – and how to keep going if you feel stuck	
Understanding why you feel as you do	
Practical problem solving	
Being assertive	
Building relationships with your baby, family and friends	
Information for families and friends – how can you offer the best support?	
Doing things that boost how you feel	
Using exercise to boost how you feel	
Helpful things you do	
Unhelpful things you do	
Anxiety and avoidance	
Noticing and changing extreme and unhelpful thinking	
Overcoming sleep problems	
Alcohol, drugs and your baby	
Understanding and using antidepressant medication	
Planning for the future	
General comments about the book	

Table 8.7 Key features of each workbook in *Overcoming teenage low mood and depression*

Workbook	Key features of that workbook
Understanding why I feel as I do	
Why bother changing?	
Doing things that make me feel good	
Using exercise to boost how I feel	
Helpful things we do	
Unhelpful things we do	
Restarting things we've avoided	
Practical problem solving	
Noticing and changing extreme and unhelpful thinking	
Being assertive	
Building relationships	
Overcoming sleep problems	
Alcohol, drugs and me	
Understanding and using antidepressant medication	
Planning for the future	
General comments about the books	

Table 8.8 Key features of each of the Little CBT Books

Resource	Key features of that resource
Write all over your bathroom mirror: And 14 other ways to get the most out of your little book	
Why do I feel so bad?	
How to fix almost everything	
Why does everything always go wrong?	
I can't be bothered doing anything	
The things you do that mess you up	
I'm not good enough: How to overcome low confidence	
Are you strong enough to keep your temper?	
10 things you can do to make you feel happier straight away	
I feel so bad I can't go on	
The Worry Box	
Enjoy your baby	
Live longer – have a heart attack	
Stop smoking in 5 minutes	
General comments about the books	

Chapter 9

Five Areas online, DVD and audio multimedia resources for low mood and stress

What you will learn

In this chapter you will learn about various Five Areas multimedia resources that address low mood, depression and anxiety. This includes:

- The **www.livinglifetothefull.com** and **www.llttfi.com** online courses.
- How the websites offer support using forums, reminder emails and newsletters.
- DVD resources: the Living Life to the Full (LLTTF) DVD and credit card resources.
- Audio resources – relaxation CDs and downloads.

Other resources aimed at helping people experiencing stress and low mood are the Living Life to the Full class (Chapter 7) and various book-based resources (Chapter 8).

Introduction

People often like to watch television or use computers as a first port of call when it comes to seeking information. Nowadays, turning to internet search engines such as Google (**www.google.com**) is a natural way for people to seek information. Figure 9.1 shows the rise in hits on **www.google.com** from 2001 to 2009 for the search terms 'self' + 'help' + 'depression'. This currently (2010) runs at over 18 million hits.

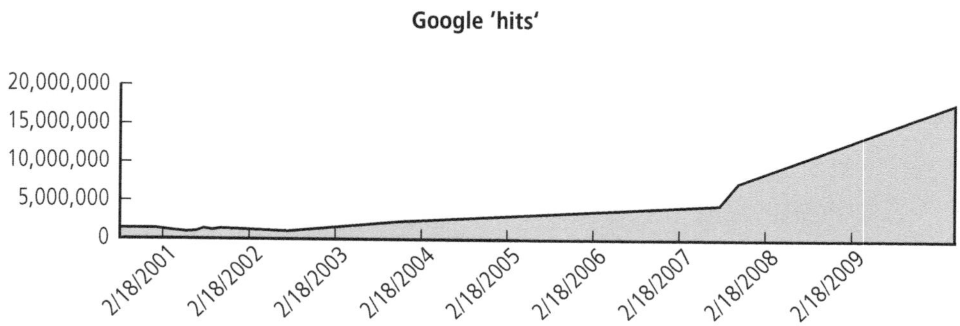

Figure 9.1 www.google.com hits for 'self' + 'help' + 'depression' (2001–10).

This chapter describes the range of multimedia-delivered Five Areas resources, and offers some practical suggestions on how to best support their use.

Advantages of multimedia-based learning

Use of multimedia resources fits in well with current lifestyles because:

- Most people now have a television and DVD player, but many barely have a book in their house or flat. CDs and DVDs are therefore usable by almost all. Not everyone wants to sit and read.
- MP3/MP4 players are owned by the majority of young people and are becoming increasingly popular among people of all ages. They can be used to store sound files (such as relaxation files) and – for some – video.
- Seeing someone else experiencing problems, learning how to overcome them and learning vicariously from this can be a powerful learning aid. Multimedia products offer the ability to watch real people who have similar problems and have used the interventions themselves.
- Computer and DVD delivered resources can act alone – or be a useful supplement to written self-help resources (see blended learning, page 138).
- Computer access via the internet provides a flexible way of delivering cognitive behavioural therapy (so-called computerised CBT or cCBT).
- cCBT is as effective as book-based CBT (note: it is *not more* effective) – so the main determinant of what is used should be based on patient choice.
- cCBT offers good value compared with other treatment options such as antidepressants.
- Many cCBT packages mix written and computerised resources. For example, the Living Life to the Full Interactive (LLTTFi) website (**www.llttfi.com**) contains handouts in PDF format to print out and accompany each session. The handouts provide a focus for note taking and reporting the results of 'putting into practice' tasks ('homework' or 'assignments').

Difference between the LLTTF website and LLTTFi website

Currently there are two Five Areas websites for people seeking help or support, to use the Five Areas approach themselves for help with low mood, or low mood and anxiety problems. There are significant differences between the sites in terms of design, aim and function (Table 9.1).

www.llttf.com (the short address for **www.livinglifetothefull.com**) is an open access, free to use website which can act as a supplement and support to the written and DVD courses. It allows the person to dip in and out when they wish – and choose to complete the available modules in any order they wish to. It provides only limited interactivity and contains effective 'talks' that supplement the various content of the book, LLTTF classes and DVD-based courses. Clinicians can register and support people through the website, and monitor progress; there is also a discussion forum for people using the website.

In contrast, the **www.llttfi.com** (the short address for **www.livinglifetothefullinteractive.com**) is a fully functioning, sophisticated and licensed (paid for) website which makes full use of multimedia and is driven by a highly intelligent support algorithm.

Table 9.1 Comparison of the LLTTF and LLTTFi websites

Features	www.livinglifetothefull.com	www.livinglifetothefull interactive.com
Short URL	**www.llttf.com**	**www.llttfi.com**
Access	Free	Licensed
Structure	User-led choice of modules – do as many or as few as they wish	Six sessions that build one on another
Intelligent content (i.e. content accessed depends on the needs of the patient)	No	Yes
Moderated forum	Yes	Yes (optional)
Automated alerts if deteriorates	No	Yes
Ability to send text reminders of tasks	No	Yes
Use of questionnaires (PHQ9/GAD7) to monitor progress	When the patient chooses to do it	At every session
Handouts to print out for each session	Yes (mostly)	Yes
Recommends use of accompanying external book (e.g. Big CBT Book, Little CBT Book or DVD)	Yes (+ session handouts to print off)	No (includes session handouts to print off)
High degree of flexibility – including ability to have service-specific versions	No	Yes
Practioner monitoring of patients they support	Yes	Yes

Key Point

A key difference between the two websites is that the Interactive site is subject to a fee (used under licence).

Focus on www.llttfi.com

This cCBT package is produced under licence by Media Innovations. The site can be used in two different ways:

- As the password-protected website at **www.lltfi.com**.
- As a specially prepared website that is produced for a specific service or clinical team. This is then either loaded onto a health service server, or held on the Media Innovations secure server. The latter has NHS-level data protection security including firewalls and physical protection of the servers.

Key features of the site (patient's perspective)

The site contains six sessions:

- Session one: What is depression?
- Session two: Getting started: creating an Action Plan.
- Session three: Identifying extreme and unhelpful thoughts.
- Session four: Challenging extreme and unhelpful thoughts.
- Session five: Learning new skills (problem solving/assertiveness).
- Session six: Planning for the future.

The site provides a high degree of reporting and monitoring of patient progress, automated alerts (for risk, an email or text alert is sent to the practitioner) and the ability for administrators to monitor the outcomes of all patients and practitioners in their service.

The online resources

If in the initial assessment the patient expresses an interest in working using computerised CBT, the practitioner can offer the LLTTF or LLTTFi resource as long as the patient has access to the internet.

> **Key Point**
>
> If using the LLTTF site, it is best for the person to also have access to the linked Little or Big CBT Books as these form the basis of the course – and the website amplifies and helps the patient get the most from these.

The next step is to help the person register 'live', set up a username, and update their initial allocated password. Then the practitioner should provide a brief overview of the Quick Start Guide for the chosen site. Versions for both sites exist and include a space to write in their personal password. Encourage the person to do this.

Next, look through the website together – identifying key elements such as the course modules, how to rate mood, and the forum. The Urgent Help button should also be identified.

The *Planner sheet* and *Review sheet* should be discussed so that the person has a clear idea of the Plan, Do, Review approach to using the modules that are outlined in greater detail in Chapter 5.

Finally, plan a date and time when the patient will do the first module. For the LLTTF website, this will include a decision as to whether to focus on completing the DVD course, LLTTF Little Books/class or the *Overcoming depression and low mood* version. To help inform this decision, when the person registers for the first time on the website, they are asked questions such as 'How do you like to learn?'

Options offered are:

- I prefer short, to-the-point information – which would suggest they use the Little CBT Books/LLTTF course.
- I prefer lots of detail and want to understand things fully – which leads to a recommendation to use the Big CBT Book version.
- I prefer television/video-style information – which leads to a recommendation to use the DVD course.

Once agreed, the patient should write on the Planner sheet the name of the first module they will work, so they are ready for the next session.

Editable paper resources and handouts

Because services are very different, we have prepared an editable handout of potential sheets about the LLTTFi package, and a description of how a typical service might support the package. This can be modified by practitioners for use in their own service and can be obtained for free by emailing training@fiveareas.com.

Typically, the package includes three components that can be helpfully included in a *Start-up resource pack envelope* that is handed, posted or emailed to the patient:

- The Quick Start Guide specific to the website
- Planner and Review sheets
- An overview of the service
- A brief biography of the support practitioner and how they will work together with the patient
- Sufficient copies of any specific outcome measures your service uses and instructions on how to complete these.

Telephone support and the online courses

Telephone support (i.e. remote/distance support) raises issues of how to help the person gain access to resources such as the Start-up resource pack/envelope described above. If there is a face to face meeting (or all support sessions are face to face) this and any linked handouts or copies of workbooks, etc. can be simply handed over at that time. However, if the support is offered by phone or email, alternative ways of providing access include:

- Post or email the Start-up resource pack/envelope.
- Post copies of workbooks or Little CBT Books.
- Provide online access to the Little CBT Books (via **www.fiveareasonline.com**) – where services can obtain a licence allowing unlimited patients to access and read the resources online. This includes the option to access the Little CBT Books and worksheets in five languages.

Using the linked worksheets

All the online courses contain handouts and worksheets. Patients should be encouraged to print these and use them to help structure their practice of what they are learning. They help the patient record information and practise repeatedly their new skills.

Other LLTTF support resources

LLTTF online newsletters

The LLTTF website offers the option to sign up for regular online newsletters that contain information, hints and tips. The patient can subscribe to or unsubscribe from these in the My Living Life area of the website when they are signed in. People can also opt out of the newsletter each time they receive it.

LLTTF regular reminder emails

It is hard to make new habits. Knowing this, the LLTTF site is designed to routinely send out once-weekly emails during the first 12 weeks of using the site. The emails include motivational encouragement – as well as specific hints and tips about how to use the website and the Planner and Review sheets.

LLTTFi manually requested reminders to login

LLTTFi has an option that allows the patient to book an email or text message to their mobile to remind them to login to the LLTTFi site at a specific time.

Data protection and privacy issues

Sometimes patients ask about the security of the data collected as they use the packages:

- LLTTF: data are physically protected. The servers are firewalled and backed up regularly. Regarding the data retained, the only personally identifiable information recorded is the person's email and postcode. Users have complete control of their own data and can choose to delete all the information they have given. To do this they can delete their entire account when logged into LLTTF.
- LLTTFi: Again high levels of data security are provided. LLTTFi records far greater amounts of personal information when people register, and this is held to NHS security standards by Media Innovations on its protected servers, or on NHS or other service servers when this is the preferred option by the service.

Key Point

All users should be encouraged to read the privacy policy and terms and conditions of the websites as these contain important information.

Using the online forums

Forums can be a helpful source of information. All registrants to LLTTF have access to a forum; this is also available on the main LLTTFi site. Forums can be used in several ways:

- To post and ask questions, make comments or to express and opinion.
- To read other people's posts and learn from them. The LLTTF forum in particular has a wealth of information on a range of topics posted with some helpful hints and tips – and there is much than can be obtained by reading them.

- A crucial role for forums is in providing support. People can receive encouragement when they are struggling, for example.

The forums are all moderated – however not every post will be read. Tell the patient to use the *Report this post* option to submit details of any inappropriate posts that need to be looked at in particular.

A note of caution

Advise patients who use the forum to read the forum rules and to be wary of swapping private details such as email addresses and home phone numbers with others. They should also be reminded that not everything posted will be true or accurate. People need to view it a bit like discussions in a pub or club: people will express their opinions; some will have greater expertise, others less so; some will be loud and assertive, others quieter and reflective. Also, like a pub or club if a person writes something onto a notice board for another person to see, many others can also see it – including people who may know the writer (if they are registered with the particular course). It is therefore wise for people to only post things they are happy for others to know.

Although the forum is only open to registered members, there is nothing to stop members copying posts and distributing them elsewhere – so for all these reasons people should be careful about what they post. To protect individuals they should only post under their public name – not their real name. If a person posts to a forum and then deeply regrets it, they can contact the forum administrators to ask for it to be edited or deleted.

Practitioner support

Throughout the chapters in this book there is a focus on guided CBT. Support helps people stay motivated and apply what they are learning. Outcomes are better as a result. Both LLTTF and LLTTFi emphasise support in several ways:

- The use of the Planner and Review sheets so the person can plan their use of the website.
- The use of newsletters and reminder emails when activated to help keep people on track.
- The forum – which itself can provide important support.
- The accompanying support of a support work/practitioner. We encourage all users of the online websites to request such support, and the LLTTF site allows a practitioner to also log in and offer a *Support Association*.

Using the LLTTF support associations

If a practitioner/supporter registers as a practitioner on LLTTF, they can offer a greater level of monitored support for their patients. Both patients and practitioners can offer an invitation to set up a support association between the two of them. This allows the practitioner to see when the patient last logged in, view mood rating scores, modules started and finished etc. This adds additional useful information that can aid support. The patient and practitioner can end the support relationship at any stage they wish. This is controlled from within their *My Living Life* area.

LLTTF DVD

The LLTTF DVD is around 40 minutes and consists of several modules:

- Introduction to the DVD (covers the Five Areas assessment model)
- Problem solving
- Building confidence
- Balanced thinking
- Unhelpful behaviours
- Sleeping better
- Healthy living
- Assertiveness

The content is produced using the well-known TV presenter Jenny Farish and includes interviews with real-life volunteers from the charity Depression Alliance Scotland.

Using the LLTTF Little CBT Books and worksheets

One issue that arises when patients use the DVD is that there are few opportunities to practise what is being presented. This problem can be addressed by linking the use of the DVD to the LLTTF colour worksheets and the Little CBT Book series. These are available as physical (printed) books and also online under licence to services who can then use the online versions with as many patients from their service as they wish. The advantage is that there is an additional structure to help people apply what they learn.

The LLTTF DVD is available in its entirety, free of charge, from **www.llttf.com** (once logged in).

Using the Planner and Review sheets

The Planner and Review sheets can again be used to underpin the practical application of what has been learned.

LLTTF DVD accompanying credit cards

The DVD is accompanied by four credit card sized cards that contain summaries of:

- The seven steps of problem solving.
- The rules of assertion.
- How to conduct a thought review.
- How to sleep better.

The cards can also be printed for free from the **www.fiveareas.com** free resources section, or purchased separately as a set of four or in bulk for use in clinical services.

Audio resources – relaxation CDs and downloads

The anxiety control training (ACT) 1 and 2 audios are available as two MP3 free downloads from the free resources section of **www.fiveareas.com**. Professionally recorded versions by Jenny Farish are also available at low cost. An audio CD with both male and female versions of the ACT is available from **www.fiveareas.com** as a single CD or in bulk for use in clinical services.

Key practice points

- Ask people how they like to learn (short, to-the-point information, lots of detail or television/video-style information) to point them to the most helpful course for them on LLTTF.
- **www.llttf.com** and **www.llttfi.com** are shortcuts to the Living Life to the Full and Living Life to the Full Interactive websites, respectively.
- To get the most from online resources the patient needs to want to use them.
- Forums can provide useful support, but the patient should be advised to take care with what is posted and to be aware that others they know may also be registered and read their posts on the forum.
- Advise people to always choose a public name that provides them with the level of anonymity they would wish.

Further reading

Williams C. (2007) *Living life to the full DVD.* Leeds: Media Innovations (ASIN: 1906330085).

PART 4

Supervision, training and service implications

Chapter 10

Case management and supervision

What you will learn

In this chapter you will learn:

- What type and level of supervision is needed or is helpful for those delivering CBT self-help interventions.
- How supervision can be delivered – and practical ways to do this using the Five Areas approach.
- Making effective use of supervision when you have 10–20, 30–40 or 60+ minutes available for supervision sessions.
- About good practice guidelines for the use of audio and video recordings.
- Using the Five Areas model for reflective practice and lifelong learning.

Incorporating supervision into services

Supervision is an important activity in the delivery of psychological therapies, and there are various ways of delivering and receiving supervision. These depend on the workplace, the type and number of patients and the availability of someone to supervise practitioners. In Latin *super* means 'over', and *vidére* means 'to watch' or 'to see'. However the true benefit of supervision in psychological therapies is not as a 'big brother' monitoring activity in terms of performance. Instead, it should be an activity that benefits practitioners and ultimately the care of the patients they look after.

Supervision involves discussing the care of the patients being supported and other aspects of clinical work with another professional or member of the team. It can be delivered individually and in groups. Usually, but not always, the person providing the supervision has more experience than the supervisee, but peer supervision provided by another person in the same area or field of work is also a popular option. The key thing is that both parties understand the aim of the clinical work and that the supervisor is also familiar with the resources and materials, and is experienced in delivering and supporting the interventions.

Key Point

If locally there is no-one suitable to supervise, look at alternative ways of accessing a supervisor, for example via the telephone.

Who can offer supervision?

Supervision can be a formal process with contracts between both parties, or may be less formal. There are many types of supervision ranging from case management and clinical skills to managerial, professional and academic. It is worth reflecting for a moment about what the aim of supervision within psychological therapies is and what would be helpful to an individual practitioner's practice.

When people are training to deliver these types of approaches a person with more clinical experiences of the intervention acting as a supervisor can ensure that all treatment options have been considered. It allows the opportunity for the trainee to discuss and reflect on the cases being seen, to raise questions, seek support and guidance, and to develop skills and confidence. However it is not only trainees who need and benefit from supervised practice, it is a lifelong activity for all practitioners. Even when therapists are fully qualified, most do and should continue to receive and benefit from supervision and reflective practice, and this is required for ongoing accreditation as an HI CBT therapist or as a low intensity practitioner by the British Association for Behavioural and Cognitive Psychotherapies (BABCP; **www.babcp.com**). Supervision is often a mandatory requirement in clinical healthcare settings.

The key thing we know about supervision is that it ensures fidelity of the evidence base of model of the treatment being delivered and can also decrease practitioner stress and burnout. To provide supervision to another person it is important that the supervisor feels adequately skilled to do so.

Supervision competencies

Competencies for the effective delivery of supervision in psychological therapies have been published (Roth and Pilling 2008) and are very useful in considering the generic and more specific competencies that are required when providing supervision in cognitive behavioural therapy (CBT)-based approaches. These are available at **www.ucl.ac.uk/clinical-psychology/WRE/competence–frameworks.htm**.

Two common models of supervision

The two main types of supervision that benefit the delivery of CBT-type approaches are case management and clinical skills. These are two very different types of supervision, with different objectives. These are usually delivered as separate sessions, for example within Increasing Access to Psychological Therapies (IAPT) services.

- In *case management*, supervisors provide an overseeing role in the care provided to patients, and help make collaborative decisions with the supervisee about the care delivered.
- In *clinical skills supervision*, the supervisor will be giving advice and acts rather like a trainer to offer skills practice and development. As a very minimum they will need to be familiar with the interventions and resources that are being used and the ways in which these are supported. They also need to be familiar with and have a strong working knowledge of the Five Areas assessment and the problem or areas of difficulty it is being used to support.

Case management

Case management is a regular review of all cases seen at scheduled intervals in care delivery – with additional supervision contacts occurring if risk increases or if the person's condition deteriorates. The focus here is on the person receiving the treatment, how they are progressing, the problem areas identified, and of course how the interventions are proceeding. In this model of supervision – which has been adopted by IAPT in England, all cases are discussed at least every four sessions. Case management does not replace the need for clinical skills supervision, as the focus and outcome of both these serve different purposes.

Clinical skills

Clinical skills supervision is an opportunity for the clinician to practise skills, learn new ideas, and discuss things they are unsure about or need more help with. This may take place individually, or in groups or in twos to allow role-play facilitation. A person may bring audio or video tapes of their practice to the session to listen to or watch and reflect on with their supervisor.

Supervision using the Five Areas approach

The Five Areas model can be used in a number of ways in supervision and reflective practice. The Five Areas assessment provides an overall summary of the patient to be discussed in supervision with your supervisor.

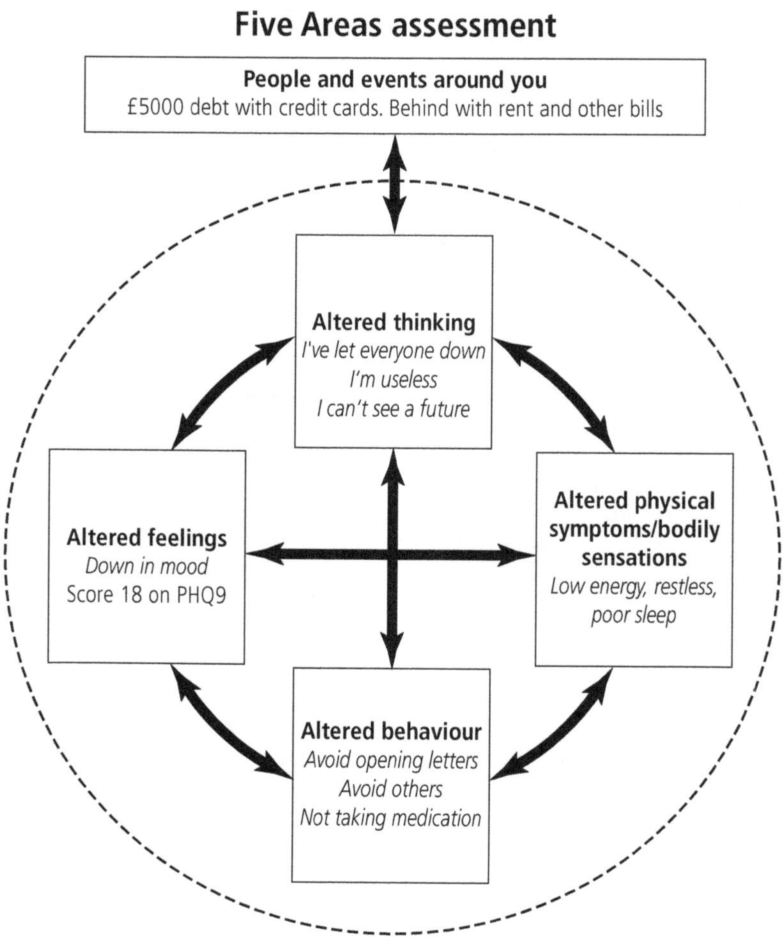

Figure 10.1 An example Five Areas summary for supervisor assessment.

The assessment can be given to the supervisor in advance of the session or at the beginning so that the patient's difficulties are clearly broken down into each of the Five Areas to see where problems lie and to identify the targets for intervention. This working problem summary can enable the supervisor to become familiar with the case. It allows a discussion of formulation and maintaining factors, and also provides a structure for further discussion.

The assessment can be also used as a quick visual summary of the treatment interventions that have been planned and how these are going to be delivered as shown in Figure 10.2. The scores of any measures used, level of risk and any other information that is important can be added to the diagram to assist in this process. This can enable the supervisor to see what has been delivered so far and the progress (or not) to date.

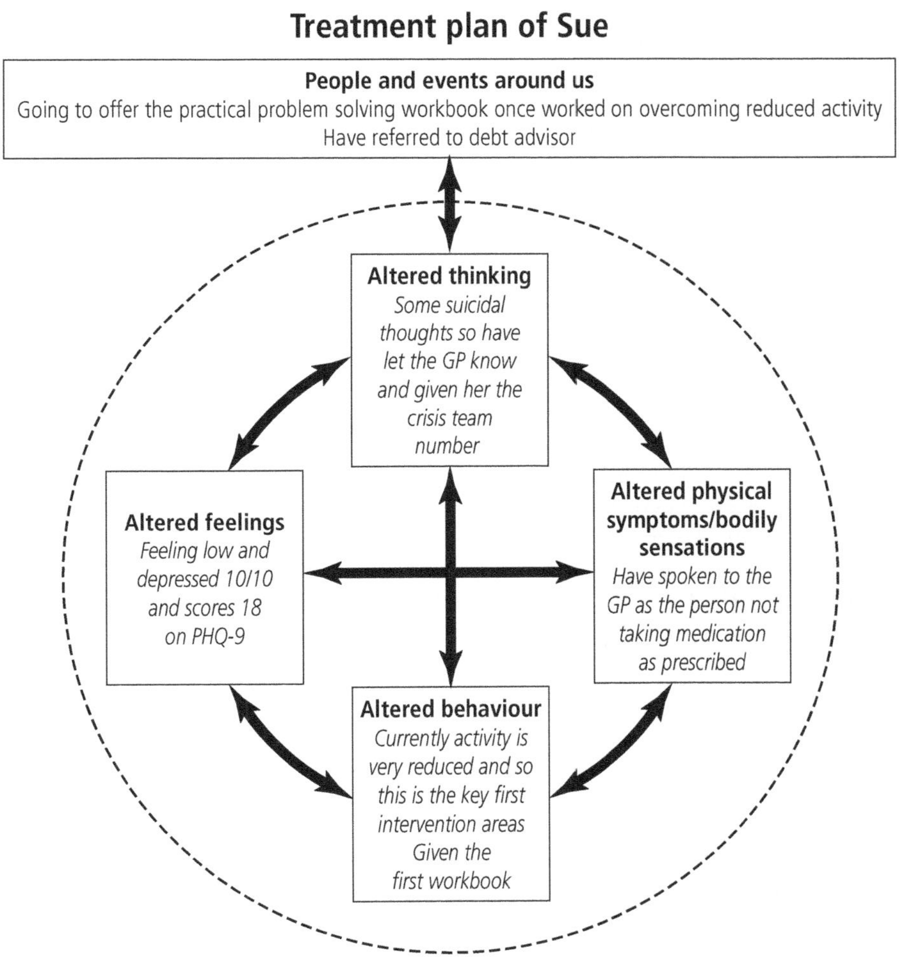

Figure 10.2 Sue's treatment plan.

The combination of the two diagrams (Figures 10.1 and 10.2) ensures the information that is required is easily at hand in supervision, in just two key documents, and that the treatment plan devised for Sue is summarised in an easy to read format. If supervision takes place over the telephone or by another method it can be helpful to email the diagrams of the cases you wish to discuss so both parties can see these during the session (protecting anonymity of course, for example, by labelling them case 1, case 2 etc.).

These two working diagrams kept in a patient's notes or file are also very useful if another practitioner or worker has to take over the case, for example if the support worker is off sick or is unable to attend the session for other reasons, or if they are moving to another service. The diagrams provide an accurate picture of the difficulties, the treatment planned and how it has gone so far.

Self-pratice/self-reflection (SP/SR)

The concept of practising CBT techniques on oneself as a practitioner and reflecting upon these as a method to improve skills and confidence is well documented in the literature (e.g. Bennett-Levy *et al.*, 2001; Bennett-Levy, 2006; Farrand *et al.*, 2010) and is used in many high and low intensity training courses. This can be a helpful method used to enhance and structure clinical skills supervision, for example with supervisees testing out an intervention on themselves that they use with patients, such as practical problem solving, or using an activity or thought diary between supervision sessions and then reflecting on this in supervision. The links to the meta-competency skill in *Guided CBT Self Help* (Skills for Health 2008) of being able to reflect on and learn from experiences (see Chapter 11 for more information about competencies). It also allows the supervisee to 'get in the shoes' of their patients and experience CBT self-help first hand, and of how demanding completing these tasks can be (even when we're not depressed or anxious).

Supervision in 10, 30 and 60 minutes

When time is short, or when the number of active cases on a caseload is high, using time effectively is important. Each added available time allows more work that builds on what can be covered in shorter sessions.

Supervision and reflective practice when only 10–20 minutes are available (or not even that)

When time is as short as this, such as may be the case in general practice settings, formal supervision may not be possible. However, there may be opportunity for shared learning and peer support that can offer useful support and guidance.

The short duration is likely to be a more informal arrangement, and would not meet the requirements of most clinical services. Some clinical skills practice could take place in this time, and if caseload size was small and the practitioner was well prepared with all relevant information, approximately five or six cases could be discussed briefly in case management supervision. Efficiency and focus can be aided by a computer-based system that contains relevant information about the cases needing case management supervision and which both the practitioner and the supervisor can see during the session.

An additional option would be *reflective practice* and *service discussion* groups. Most people in any setting would be able to identify 10–20 minutes that they could use to provide a level of supervisory or reflective practice activities during a week or month. This could be delivered, for example, in weekly team meetings; 10–20 minutes could be set aside for a case presentation, providing shared learning for peers, and an opportunity to discuss any areas of a patient's care that it would be useful to have more opinions on, or using SP/SR to reflect on interventions, perhaps face to face or via the use of online blogs (e.g. Farrand *et al.*, 2010).

Supervision or reflective practice when 30–40 minutes are available

In 30–40 minutes there is significantly more time available to explore the case management of patients on a practitioner's caseload, and to work on developing clinical skills. Thirty minutes of clinical skills supervision on a one to one basis with the supervisor would allow time for practising assessment and treatment session skills, and support methods, and would reflect the time often used in actual clinical sessions with patients. Such supervision could be delivered in a group so that all people attending can benefit from the discussion and skills practice.

Role-play can take place between supervisor and supervisee to practise techniques, questioning style or support. If two or more people are being supervised at once, role-play can take place between the supervisees with the supervisor observing and giving feedback.

Case management within 30–40 would give the opportunity for approximately 10–12 cases to be discussed if all information was prepared or available within the supervision session, for example by having access to the notes or computerised data management programme. However, this would still be considered a relatively short session and would not meet the requirements of some services, for example IAPT services.

Supervision or reflective practice when 60 minutes (or more) are available

This amount of time is the usual duration of both a clinical skills and a case management supervision session, and the amount of time that is a minimum requirement in most services, for example within IAPT settings.

Group 60-minute clinical skills sessions can focus on particular interventions or a full assessment role-play, and in case management even with a high caseload number all the cases that would require review are likely to be covered in the time.

In traditional CBT service settings outside primary care, clinical skills supervision often only occurs once a month, but in most psychological therapy services this would occur at least fortnightly. In higher intensity CBT, the clinical skills focus would typically allow the discussion of one to three cases in a one-hour session.

Using audio and video

There are significant benefits in clinical skills supervision of having the opportunity to bring along audio or video of live sessions. The patient should provide informed writen consent before the practitioner can record with audio/video, and a copy of this signed consent form should be placed in the patient's file. They should be asked to agree to this verbally on any recording so it can be heard by the supervisor. They should also be reminded that they can withdraw consent at any time, and be informed about the purpose of the recording and how long it will be kept and when it will be disposed of. They can withdraw consent at any time.

Such records are often now kept on electronic devices such as MP3 players. These may be easily lost or stolen, so thought needs to be given as to how files will be labelled and protected. It is good practice to encrypt such folders or USB drives. Patient names should not be written onto audio CDs or DVD disks in case they are lost. All such files remain as part of the clinical record. However, it is often the case that files are lost out of notes, so it can be argued they are best destroyed when finished with.

Patient use of supervision materials

A great advantage of recording audio live in a face to face session is that not only can it be used in supervision, but also the patient can be given a copy to listen to again at home. The main downside of this is that it can take significant time to cut an audio disk.

Key Point

When recording telephone support sessions, the use of a digital voice recorder is essential. A device called a TP7 by the manufacturer Olympus is easily obtainable at low cost on the internet and can be used to provide high quality recordings. Note: it is illegal to record a telephone conversation without consent in the UK.

Example: Good practice guidelines for the recording of audio/video

(from the General Medical Council; see **www.gmc-uk.org/guidance/ethical_guidance/making_audiovisual.asp**)

Practitioners should:

'Seek permission to make the recording and get consent for any use or disclosure.

Give patients adequate information about the purpose of the recording when seeking their permission.

Ensure that patients are under no pressure to give their permission for the recording to be made.

Stop the recording if the patient asks you to, or if it is having an adverse effect on the consultation or treatment.

Do not participate in any recording made against a patient's wishes.

Ensure that the recording does not compromise patients' privacy and dignity.

Do not use recordings for purposes outside the scope of the original consent for use, without obtaining further consent.

Make appropriate secure arrangements for storage of recordings'.

In addition, 'Before the recording, you must ensure that patients:

1. Understand the purpose of the recording, who will be allowed to see it – including names if they are known – the circumstances in which it will be shown, whether copies will be made, the arrangements for storage and how long the recording will be kept.
2. Understand that withholding permission for the recording to be made, or withdrawing permission during the recording, will not affect the quality of care they receive.
3. Are given time to read explanatory material and to consider the implications of giving their written permission. Forms and explanatory material should not imply that permission is expected. They should be written in language that is easily understood. If necessary, translations should be provided.

After the recording, you must ensure that:

1. Patients are asked if they want to vary or withdraw their consent to the use of the recording.
2. Recordings are used only for the purpose for which patients have given consent.
3. Patients are given the chance, if they wish, to see the recording in the form in which it will be shown.
4. Recordings are given the same level of protection as medical records against improper disclosure.
5. If a patient withdraws or fails to confirm consent for the use of the recording, the recording is not used and is erased as soon as possible.'

A format for low intensity supervision to suit low intensity practice

Figure 10.3 provides a structure for organising supervision of workers using low intensity models that is currently used in Five Areas services in Glasgow. Here there are far too many patients to allow discussion about each patient at every supervision session. The structure

Patient Name **ID No**
Date referred first self-referred

Baseline/recruitment Date first seen: Date discussed:	**4-week review** Date due: Date discussed:	**8-week review (final review)** Date due: Date discussed:
Problem statement: Treatment plan agreed: Signed:	Problem statement: Treatment plan agreed: Signed:	Problem statement: Treatment plan agreed: Signed:

ADDITIONAL CASE REVIEWS

Active risk, deterioration, missed contact, other concern? Date due: Date discussed:	**Active risk, deterioration, missed contact, other concern?** Date due: Date discussed:	**Active risk, deterioration, missed contact, other concern?** Date due: Date discussed:
Treatment plan agreed: Signed:	Treatment plan agreed: Signed:	Treatment plan agreed: Signed:

Risk/deterioration/non-contact/drop-out: discuss that week. **Active risk**: discuss that day. **Active risk (suicidality)**: inform supervisor/clinical lead and respond using service standard risk management protocol.

Figure 10.3 Single patients review/action sheets.

Name/Participant ID	Baseline review	4-week review	8-week/final review	Red flag?
Name: ID: Date entered:	Date due: Date done: Initials:	Date due: Date done: Initials:	Date due: Date done: Initials:	Date due: Date done: Initials:
Name: ID: Date entered:	Date due: Date done: Initials:	Date due: Date done: Initials:	Date due: Date done: Initials:	Date due: Date done: Initials:
Name: ID: Date entered:	Date due: Date done: Initials:	Date due: Date done: Initials:	Date due: Date done: Initials:	Date due: Date done: Initials:
Name: ID: Date entered:	Date due: Date done: Initials:	Date due: Date done: Initials:	Date due: Date done: Initials:	Date due: Date done: Initials:
Name: ID: Date entered:	Date due: Date done: Initials:	Date due: Date done: Initials:	Date due: Date done: Initials:	Date due: Date done: Initials:
Name: ID: Date entered:	Date due: Date done: Initials:	Date due: Date done: Initials:	Date due: Date done: Initials:	Date due: Date done: Initials:

Figure 10.4 Total caseload overview sheets.

therefore provides a focused, short and structured solution to this problem. It aims to balance the need to review patients at set time points (baseline, one month and end of treatment – often but not always at about eight weeks). In addition, any patient experiencing difficulties is discussed ('red-flagged') for more urgent discussion when there is:

- Active risk: check each support contact.
- Deterioration: worsening objective scores or statements of such.
- Missed contact: i.e. not rearranged.
- Other concern: anything the supporting practitioner is worried about.

Using the Five Areas model for reflective practice and facilitating lifelong learning

The Five Areas model can be used as a summary and structure for reflection on a practitioner's own practice and skills at any time. Busy working or home lives means stress can build up, especially when learning new skills or when the demands placed on people are high. Practitioners are also human beings and at times may find colleagues, a family member or a particular person they are working with difficult.

At times a practitioner may become anxious about the interventions they are delivering, or indeed any other aspect of their work. Completing a Five Areas reflective diagram of their own at these times is a useful way of being able to stop, think and reflect, and look at ways in which it may be helpful or unhelpful to respond. This can also be useful to aid reflective practice after sessions that have gone well, or perhaps that did not go as well as planned.

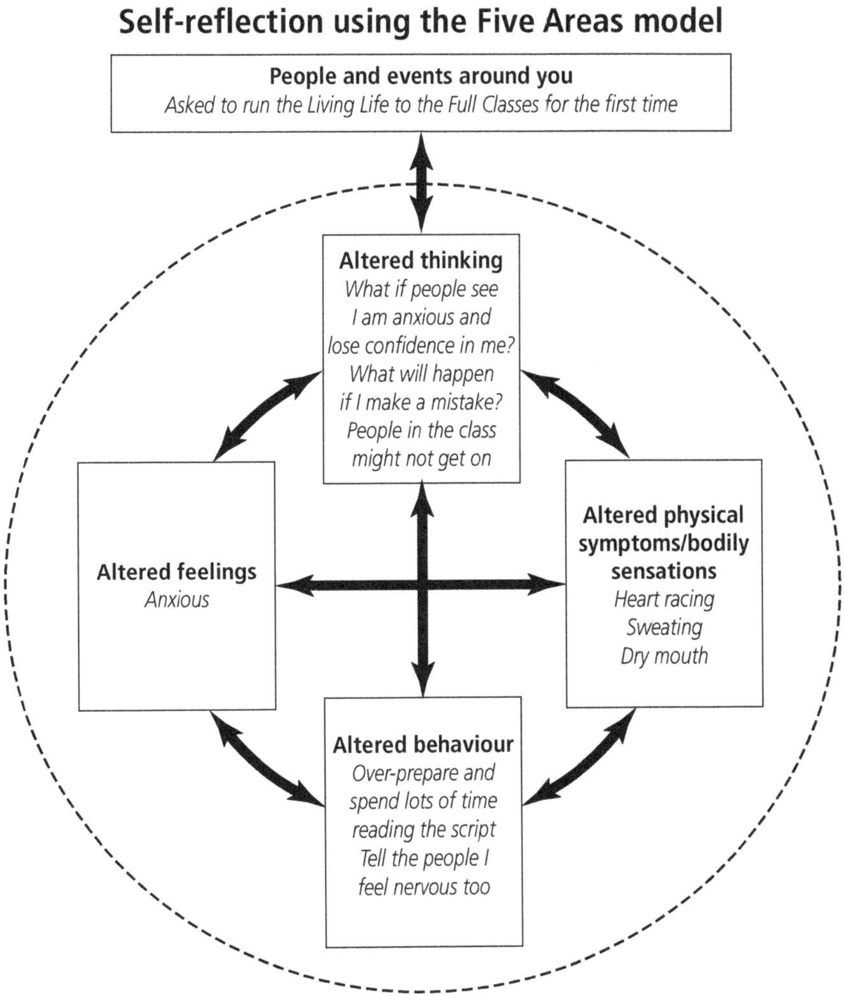

Figure 10.5 Self-reflection using the Five Areas model.

This may then be something that the practitioner can work through alone, or something that they can take to their clinical skills supervision for further advice and guidance. The diagram can also be a very good way of structuring reflection when undertaking SP/SR, for example by completing a diagram to reflect on the process of completing an activity diary and noting thoughts and feelings when doing this.

Key practice points

- Case management and clinical supervision are two of the most used forms of supervision.
- Self-practice/self-reflection (SP/SR) of techniques is a valuable tool for use in training and supervision to benefit clinical practice.
- Low intensity working requires adjustments to the traditional supervision framework.

- Case management is generally more suited to low intensity working.
- Making audio or video tapes of consultations for use in supervision/case management has particular ethical and good practice issues that require a consistent and planned approach.
- Treatment guidelines confirm the need for regular supervision to help practitioners stay faithful to the treatment model and offer effective interventions.

Reference

Bennett-Levy, J. (2006). Therapists skills: a cognitivie model of their acquisition and refinement. *Behavioural and Cognitive Psychotherapy* **34**: 57–78.

Bennett-Levy J, Turner F, Beaty T, Smith M, Paterson B, Farmer S. (2001) The value of self-practice of cognitive therapy techniques and self-reflection in the training of cognitive therapists. *Behavioural and Cognitive Psychotherapy* **29**: 203–220.

Farrand P, Perry J, Linsley S. (2010) Enhancing Self practice/self reflection (SP/SR) approach to cognitive behaviour training through the use of reflection blogs. *Behavioural and Cognitive Psychotherapy*, doi:10.1017/S1352465810000238.

Richards D, Chellingsworth M, Hope R, Turpin G, Whyte M. (2010) *Reach Out. National programme supervisor materials to support the delivery of training for psychological wellbeing practictioners delivering low intensity interventions.* London: Rethink. Available at: **www.iapt.nhs.uk/wp-content/uploads/supervisors-manualfeb15.pdf**.

Skills for Health. (2008) See **www.ucl.ac.uk/clinical-psychology/CORE/CBT-Framework.htm**.

Further reading

Richards D, Chellingsworth M, Hope R, Turpin G, Whyte M. (2010). *Reach Out: National programme supervisor materials to support the delivery of training for psychological wellbeing practitioners delivering low intensity interventions.* London: Rethink. Available at: **www.iapt.nhs.uk/wp-content/uploads/supervisors-manual-feb15.pdf**.

Roth AD, Pilling S. (2008) A competence framework for the supervision of psychological therapies. Available at: **www.ucl.ac.uk/clinical-psychology/CORE/ competence_frameworks.htm**.

Chapter 11

Training and supporting practitioners in using the Five Areas approach

> **What you will learn**
>
> **In this chapter you will learn about:**
>
> - Why training in using the Five Areas approach can help.
> - How to make what is taught essential, i.e. how to 'sell' the idea of locally delivered training to potential attendees and to funders.
> - Delivering training that is relevant, varied and interesting.
> - How the Plan, Do, Review model can be used as a training tool.
> - Ways of evaluating changes in knowledge, skills and attitudes.
> - How to make training 'stick', so that people continue to use what they have learned after the training.

Why training in low intensity working matters

It is widely accepted that patient outcomes in high intensity cognitive behavioural therapy (CBT) for depression are maximised if the practitioner is trained, supervised and works using a manualised model (NICE, 2009). We also know that over 95 per cent of accredited practitioners use guided CBT on a regular basis (Keeley *et al.*, 2002). However, large-scale surveys of practitioners accredited by the British Association for Behavioural and Cognitive Psychotherapies (BABCP; **www.babcp.com**) show that few have been trained in how to introduce and support CBT self-help resources. Those who have been trained feel more confident in working in this way, and also have a more positive view of the guided CBT approach (Keeley *et al.*, 2002; Whitfield and Williams, 2004). It should not be assumed that working in LI ways is 'straightforward' or 'commonsense'. Like HI interventions, training and using a clear structure will improve outcomes. We know that guided CBT interventions can be effectively delivered by practitioners who have not undergone extensive psychotherapy training (Williams *et al.*, 2010)

The focus of this chapter is therefore on how to structure and deliver training that it is relevant, targeted, attractive and useful. Such training needs to build competencies in delivering guided CBT effectively.

Competency frameworks in using CBT self-help

Training has long since moved on from a situation where practitioners just attended classes or simply had to pass a written examination. Both low and high intensity CBT courses have increasingly acknowledged the need to assess competencies, i.e. whether the person can adequately deliver the skills taught in everyday practice outside the classroom environment. Competency frameworks have been published for both high and low intensity working by Skills for Health in England (Skills for Health, 2008a,b). The competencies for guided CBT are available online from **www.ucl.ac.uk/clinical-psychology/WRE/CBT_Framework.htm#map**.

The competency frameworks is a very uselful document. It outlines in detail the competencies required for the delivery of guided CBT self-help and structures these in the following domains: generic compentencies, establishing a framework for CBT self-help, basic CBT competencies, and meta-compentencies. This is intended to help users see how the various activities fit together. It is not a hierarchial model, with some domains being more important or requiring more skill than others. Any intervention at high or low intensity level requires clinicians to bring together knowledge and skills from across the domains.

In Box 11.1 we have also provided the reader with further specific competencies which build on these but are specifically related to the delivery of the Five Areas model.

Box 11.1 Competencies in introducing and supporting CBT and self-help

Generic practitioner competencies (non-specific factors)

Be able to:

- Build a warm, trusting and encouraging therapeutic relationship.
- Communicate clearly using accessible and simple to understand concepts/ language.
- Outline a model of safe working involving regular risk assessments – and be able to respond according to a written risk management plan.
- Educate the patient how and when to seek help if they deteriorate.
- Use short rating questionnaires to monitor outcomes, alert to deterioration and identify active risk.
- Jointly agree with the patient how much and what type of follow-up will be offered if the patient disengages.

Generic self-help delivery

Be able to:

- Describe key elements of the evidence base of the guided CBT/cCBT model.
- Identify whether the person wishes to use guided CBT.
- Assess whether the person can use CBT self-help.

- Agree which self-help format is appropriate for that particular person at this time.
- Identify what type and amount of support they prefer (face to face, telephone, class-based or email/online), how frequent the support contacts will be, and how long the support sessions should be.
- Explain the need for a clear plan to use the self-help resources – and introduce the Plan, Do Review model based around using the Planner and Review Sheets.
- Use protocol-driven support scripts – while communicating these in ways that engage the individual patient.
- Problem solve difficulties the patient experiences in using/applying the self-help resources.

Specific Five Areas resource delivery

Practitioners should work with patients to:

- Describe the Five Areas model and its components and how they link together as a vicious circle.
- Carry out a Five Areas summary of key problems and strengths/resources.
- Use their own Five Areas summary to explain symptoms to a patient.
- Collaboratively identify targets for change using the Five Areas summary and 'sell' the idea that making changes in any area is worthwhile.
- Negotiate specific short-term targets for change – within a context of medium and longer changes relevant to the person.
- Be familiar with the range of Five Areas written and computerised forms of self-help used within the service so that individual workbooks and other resources can be identified and introduced to the patient when needed.
- Describe the key elements of the vicious circles of reduced activity, avoidance and unhelpful behaviours, and the basis for breaking such circles in a planned way.
- Provide an overview of the seven steps to problem solving for tackling reduced activity, overcoming unhelpful behaviours and reducing avoidance.
- Describe the impact of unhelpful thinking styles and help patients identify unhelpful thinking styles using the thinking styles checklist.
- Be able to describe the components of the thought investigation approach with reference to the self-help resources.
- Be able to describe the components of the thought challenge approach with reference to the self-help resources.

The above checklist also provides a useful resource for planning training and supervision in using the Five Areas approach. See also Chapter 6, which contains a summary of protocolised support scripts and low intensity adherence checklists.

Building on existing competencies

It is important to realise that for existing qualified practitioners working in roles across the health and social care workforce, and for others (e.g. in the voluntary sector), many of these skills of engagement and support will already be there. This means that training isn't starting from scratch, but instead builds on *prior learning* and experiences.

Most practice nurses, general practitioners, health visitors, psychiatrists, psychologists, counsellors and occupational therapists (i.e. almost everyone based in health or social services settings!) currently use handouts, educational and other resources with the people they help and support. They also have existing structures of working, engaging and communicating. The skills to introduce and support CBT self-help do not therefore require them to undergo a wholesale change in the way they work.

Having realistic training goals

Following a few specific principles concerning how to introduce and support self-help (e.g. the Plan, Do, Review model) in addition to the competencies already in place can make a big difference. Just as patients are not expected to change everything all at once, similarly with practitioners in training, the key would be to have different sizes and shapes of training that can slowly introduce specific changes that make a big difference in the practitioner's working practices. For the practitioners themselves, their training needs will depend on their current practice, prior learning and the number of training sessions available (or that can be attended).

Making it essential: how to 'sell' the idea of locally delivered training

Training often is one of the first areas to be cut when there are limited budgets. It is important then in creating any sustainable model of training to involve commissioners and key local training bodies such as locals NHS training committees or the workforce deanery. Key points that can help 'sell' the value of such training are:

- **National initiatives** and the need for local services to deliver treatment such as CBT self-help identified by reviews such as those of NICE (2007, 2009) and the Scottish Intercollegiate Guidelines Network (SIGN, 2010).
- **Local initiatives** such as the need to address waiting lists and build service capacity. This can include how the training will address findings of a local *training needs assessment/survey*. This can help provide evidence of a 'ground-up' call for the training that addresses local as well as national needs.
- **Arguments based on improved local patient care** with higher capacity, locally based, high quality service delivery using an evidence-based model. This can be linked with arguments concerning capacity.
- **Sustainability:** A concern when training is delivered is what will happen if a member of staff leaves the role and their replacement needs training. The skills learned can be retained by having local 'champions' or trainers to keep the work going after the initial training investment. A 'training the trainers' cascade-style model can work well where one or two identified local practitioners can continue to train others. See the short description of the SPIRIT training course in Part 5.

- **Meeting the continued professional development (CPD) and workforce development needs of the service:** This is a worthy aim, but as noted above, training budgets are often a first target when financial squeezes occur.
- **Economic arguments** such as used by Layard (2006) that services can more than save their own costs by introducing stepped access to CBT approaches. However, in our experience such arguments are not seen as especially relevant at a local level, as money from helping people back to work comes from different budgets from those that fund health service training.
- **Using the results of pilots:** Finally, establishing that what is being taught is high quality and can be delivered in a consistent way is important. So, piloting the training programme with a small number of people, obtaining feedback and writing training reports that are widely distributed can be helpful to get support to role this out more widely.
- Finally, 'pitching' the idea to key decision makers is essential.

Example

If, say, 200 staff members are trained in using CBT self-help and they all support just five people each using the approach in the next year, it means 1000 people are offered this approach etc.

The same calculation can be made to show even higher numbers if you also include the increased numbers of people who can be supported if there is a move to offer even a small proportion of patients (e.g. 25 per cent) a low intensity intervention. So instead of one patient taking say 12 hours of therapy they might receive just four hours. This allows up to three times as many people to receive full 'doses' of support for the equivalent time.

By using these various calculations the positive impact of training can be summarised. There are online workforce calculators (e.g. **www.iapt.nhs.uk/wp-content/uploads/2009/03/ct_2.xls**) that can help calculate caseload capacity for different types of worker. However, typically a high intensity practitioner will have a current caseload of around 20, compared with an average of 60+ for a low intensity practitioner.

Hopefully, bringing together the variety of different threads above will make a compelling case for training as the answer to the commissioner's or manager's needs.

How to make training content relevant, varied and interesting

Training that depends on simply slide after slide of information can be quite boring – and crucially runs the risk of not teaching any key competencies/practical skills. To teach practical skills, a variety of approaches can be used:

- **Small group discussion**: 'How would you describe the vicious circle of reduced activity in words that are really understandable?' 'How could you use this in your next clinic?' 'What difficulties might lead someone to forget to read the workbook over the next week?'

- **Video presentation and discussion**: 'What did you see on the video that were good/ poorer examples of communication?', 'What seemed to work well when they reviewed the last week?', 'Let's stop the tape just now – how could the practitioner help the person just after they said "I'll never get better?"' The key here is not just to watch video, but to **interact** with it, making comments, judgments and decisions – in a constructive way.
- **Structured practice and role-play**: Role-play sometimes has a bad reputation as 'embarrassing'. Many practitioners prefer to avoid it if they can. However in our experience it is often a powerful way of facilitating change. In Glasgow we use trained actors and pick out core skills in introducing and reviewing the use of self-help resources using a longer formal role-play. Even if budgets will not run to this, people can work in threes – one as practitioner, one as patient, and the third as a constructive observer – and rotate round these roles.
- Self-practice/self-reflection: As outlined in Chapter 10, when training practictioners can benefit greatly from practising the interventions on themselves, and with peers between training sessions, and reflecting upon the process of what went well, what didn't go so well and how this can be improved – for example, using an activity diary for a week, or using the practical problem solving steps on a practical problem in their own life. For maximum benefit this needs to be planned as set tasks directed by the trainers.

Being effective *before* the training session

We usually recommend that two trainers co-lead training sessions. This allows one to present the material and the other to reflect, observe and comment as needed. They can swap over from time to time to share the load.

It is well worthwhile meeting before the presentation with sufficient time to:

- Create a **training plan** with clear goals/aims and objectives. When creating a training session, ensure that it will be interesting, will address the needs of the trainees, provides a varied mix of information and skills practice and is competency based.
- Set up the room in the way that meets the trainer's training goals. For example, if people will be discussing things in small groups, sitting people in threes to fives around small tables works far better than having people sitting across inflexible lecture-style rows of seats. This also means it is worth thinking about what rooms to book for training some time in advance. If there isn't the flexibility for this, use what is there, but don't be afraid to rearrange the room if needed.
- Prepare all handouts, certificates of attendance and other resources needed in advance. Photocopiers have a bad habit of breaking down on the day when needed. Check the equipment is working, e.g. that laptops can 'talk' to projectors (see *A few notes on technology* later in this chapter).
- If using video from a laptop – it is worthwhile using external powered laptop speakers, otherwise some attendees may not be able to hear the video in larger audiences.
- Find out if there is a local technician, and note their number in case there is a problem using the equipment. They can advise on the phone even if they can't come out to help.

A format for delivering training

Someone once summarised effective training as involving: *Tell 'em, Tell 'em* and *Tell 'em*. This means:

- Tell those attending what you're going to teach on (i.e. the aims of the session).
- Tell them (i.e. deliver the main content of the session).
- At the end, provide a summary/review of the key points that were covered so that you tell 'em what you have told 'em.

This highlights again the need for specific training goals at each session.

Being effective during the training session

Once the training has started, there are a number of ways of making it interesting and effective:

- Agree 'training rules' at the start of a session or course. In this the trainer jointly agrees with attendees certain basic rules. This might include rules that apply to the *trainers* (e.g. starting and finishing on time, making sure everyone has an opportunity to contribute, trainers not picking on people etc.) and for the *attendees* (e.g. coming back from breaks on time, and an expectation to try things out, let everyone contribute if they wish etc.). People can be reminded of the agreed rules later in the training if issues arise that need to be addressed (see Overcoming three common problems in training, pages 180–181).
- If offering training over a number of sessions, have separate aims/objectives for each session.
- Pay attention to the content of each session to mix fact-giving with more interactive and skills-based discussions and tasks based around practical demonstrations of competency.
- Avoid information overload with too much information on too many slides.
- Pitch information at the right level of the audience – and make the content relevant to their needs.
- Only ask one question at a time – to avoid confusion.
- Why/what/where/when/how type questions (i.e. open questions) are helpful to get people discussing things and avoid straight yes/no answers.
- Remember to always gather – and look at – feedback of the session to see if you have met your training goals. Feedback forms should ideally be short – and it is worth making an effort to collect them. One effective approach is to swap properly completed forms for attendance certificates at the end of the day.

A few notes on technology

A trainer should be confident in the use of the technology widely used in presentations and teaching when delivering training. It is easy to become besotted with PowerPoint's facilities to have information swirling across the screen etc. but this can be overdone.

A basic knowledge of how to connect a laptop to a projector, toggling the video output so the image projects properly, will be essential at some point in training work.

Most laptops have three settings:

- Laptop screen only.
- Projector output only.

Key Point

It is better to focus on getting the content right than on using all the available 'flashier' aspects of PowerPoint. Try not to have more than four to six lines of text per slide: use a large font that is easily read (such as Arial). Make sure the background and text colours provide sufficient contrast to be easily read. Text that is too small to read easily just irritates people and is best avoided. Also avoid green colour for text or underlining things, as this can cause problems for people with certain learning difficulties such as dyslexia.

- Dual laptop screen and projector output – this is the setting that is desired in most situations.

A trainer can usually toggle between the three settings by pressing simultaneously the Function key and (usually) either the F5 or F6 keys (whichever has a picture of a computer monitor above it). Remember to wait a few seconds to see how it alters what is projected before repeating.

Remember:

- There are often a large number of wires in the projector bag. The only two needed are the power supply and the so-called VGA wire which transfers the video signal. This should run from the laptop VGA socket to the computer-in socket on the projector and can be usually screwed in place by hand to make sure there is a good connection.
- When it is all working, the trainer can blank out the screen during a PowerPoint presentation by pushing the B button – and un-blank it by pushing it again. The same applies to whiting out the screen using the W button.

Move through the presentation by pressing the space bar or Enter key to move forwards, or the arrow keys to move backwards and forwards.

If the technology won't work, shut everything down. Switch on the projector first, wait 60 seconds, then switch on the laptop – having made sure all the wires are correctly connected first. If it still won't work ring for the technician! It's always handy to have an interactive activity that does not rely upon the projector and laptop planned for times like this, so that the training group can continue to learn and enjoy the training until the problem is rectified.

Playing audio on laptops

A number of things can affect whether audio plays from a laptop. The most important thing is to make sure that the mute button hasn't been switched on by accident or by another person who used the laptop previously. To check this, look at the bottom right of the laptop screen for a speaker icon. If it isn't there, look for an arrow in that area and click it – this should allow you to see the speaker icon. Double click the speaker icon – this will open the Volume control. If there is a black tick in the Mute all box, then unclick it. Also make sure all the sliders are pulled towards the top of their slider bars – especially the left hand one addressing volume. Once complete, click the red X at the top right of the Volume control box to close it.

Next, make sure any external powered speakers are connected to the correct output socket (there are usually two – one for microphones (wrong) and one for headphones (right)). Check the power switch on the speakers is on (a red or green power light should be seen if it is powered) and that the volume on the volume control on the speakers is turned up. Then play the video or audio source – and you should hear audio. If not, then again ask a technician.

How to use the Plan, Do, Review model during training

The Planner sheet and separate Review sheet used in the Plan, Do, Review patient support model also provide an excellent structure for use in training. For example, the Planner sheet can be added as a regular feature towards the end of any training session. It allows attendees to choose just one or two things that they have learned and plan what they will do to build on the session they have just completed. The structure helps them both to generate a specific plan to put learning into practice, and also to predict any possible blocks that may occur. This serves a dual purpose. First, it helps them create a clear plan that is more likely to be effective. Second, it mimics the structure they themselves will be using with their patients in line with the notion of self-practice/self-reflection (SP/SR) as outlined in Chapter 10.

The attendee is also asked to complete the Review sheet and bring it along for discussion at the start of the next training session. If the training is a one-off session, then they can instead be provided with the Review sheet to take away and complete at an appropriate time later that week after they have done (or not done) the task they had planned.

Thus using the sheets provides powerful experiential learning of quite how difficult it is for anyone – practitioner or patient – to plan changes in their life. The insights gained will help inform the practitioner how to introduce and support their own patients in using the self-help approach and forms part of the SP/SR model of skill development in CBT (above and Chapter 10).

Ways of evaluating changes in knowledge, skills and attitudes

Regular use of feedback forms should be a basic feature of all training. In addition, there is the opportunity to evaluate gains in knowledge, skills and attitudes.

Evaluating knowledge gains

A number of techniques can be used including:

- **Self-rated knowledge**: e.g. by using Likert type (line) rating scales (e.g. rated 1, not at all to 7, a great deal, etc.). A problem is that self-rated and objectively rated evaluations do not always correspond. In other words, people often overestimate their own knowledge.
- **Objectively rated knowledge**: e.g. by using multiple-choice questions, or other forms of evaluation such as extended matched questions (EMQs) where a variety of responses (some correct and some not) are provided in list form – from which the practitioner chooses the correct answer to a number of questions.

Evaluating attitude gains

Various approaches can be used including reflective journals, class based discussion, and, again, the use of Likert-style questions.

Evaluating skills gains

- **Self-rated skills**: Likert type (line) rating scales can be used. Again, using this approach alone is likely to lead to an inaccurate summary as people may overestimate their skills.
- **Objectively rated knowledge**: This can include the use of video tapes/DVDs where the task is to encourage the person to pick out symptoms, create a formulation (Five Areas assessment) or create a vicious circle (e.g. of reduced activity) that summarises the case being shown. An alternative is to use actors who present a consistent (scripted) presentation. This can be marked using an objective structured clinical evaluation (OSCE) framework. Here, a single actor is interviewed by the trainee in front of a trainer who rates the knowledge, skills and attitudes using a standardised mark sheet. This can be recorded on to a DVD or videotape to allow the trainee to reflect upon their performance using a measure such as the one outlined in Table 11.1. Three example OSCEs and their mark schemes are available for download from **www.fiveareas.com**.

Classically, practitioners undergoing high intensity CBT training on postgraduate CBT courses (such as those in Oxford, London, Newcastle, Nottingham, Dundee and South of Scotland) are asked to tape or digitally record/video sessions. The tapes are then listened to with the supervisor and rated using a standardised rating scale such as the Cognitive Therapy Rating Scale Revised (CTS-R, Blackburn *et al.*, 2001). This systematically rates the therapeutic relationship, the structure of the session (e.g. agenda setting, review of homework, session summary and collaborative homework setting), and content (formulation driven, CBT interventions and use of Socratic questions) of the session.

An equivalent rating scale developed for use in guided CBT settings is shown in Table 11.1. The purpose is to again to evaluate these same three areas but in ways that are appropriate in low intensity working:

- The therapeutic relationship.
- The structure of the session.
- The content (focused on facilitating the use of guided CBT).

(These same areas form the basis in expanded form of the protocolised support script described in Chapter 6.)

Table 11.1 Guided CBT Rating Scale (GCRS, Williams 2009)

		Not (0)	Part (1)	Fully (2)
1	**Agenda setting/structure**			
a	Collaborative agenda: agree what will be covered in the session			
b	The presence of a focus and clear structure to the session			
c	Avoids straying into offering general 'therapy' outside the remit of the intervention			
2	**Collaborative relationship**			
a	Encourages the patient to participate fully through questioning, summarising/checking understanding shared problem-solving and decision making, etc.			
b	Adequate time for the patient to answer questions			
3	**Communication skills**			
a	The patient was put at ease by the practitioner's verbal skills			
b	Showed warmth, empathy and genuineness			
c	Used open and closed questions appropriately to help the patient to learn			
d	Checking/clarified and summarised what was said			
e	Pacing – so that the session doesn't seem rushed			
4a	**Covered key areas in the protocol – start of session 1**			
a	The aim of treatment approach/what you will learn			
b	How we will work together (check names/escape word)			
c	Risk assessment/management			
d	Planner task that takes key aspects of the session into the week			
4b	**Covered key areas in the protocol – other session(s)**			
a	Explore how easy it has been to use the materials between sessions (homework)			
b	Review experience of using the materials (what has been learned? what's gone well/not so well? has it been helpful/unhelpful?)			
c	Risk assessment/management			
d	Planner task that takes key aspects of the session into the week			
5	**Ending**			
a	Check what has been learned: Has new learning/understanding about the problem occurred?			
b	Homework task has been set (e.g. continue to use the materials)			

Overall judgment of session:	Satisfactory	Unsatisfactory
Session delivery		
Content		
Comments:		

Making it stick: using locally based practice and review sessions

A key issue in training is whether any training gains are sustained, and crucially are they used in practice? This can be evaluated by using follow-up questionnaires and interviews to ask practitioners to what extent they are:

- Using the workbooks (e.g. how many given out this week).
- Completing the Five Areas assessments.
- Giving the patient a copy of the Five Areas assessment.

From a service-wide perspective, it is possible to record CBT self-help interventions as an intervention on electronic patient records (e.g. by adding a dropdown menu to allow a record of the workbooks, DVD, etc. that are used). We have also found that adding the Five Areas assessment as a routine part of the admission paperwork in inpatient settings has been one of the largest factors leading to its use in Glasgow.

Our findings of the general mental health workforce show that the greater the number of sessions attended, the greater is the use of the collaborative problem-focused clinical assessment approach ($r = 0.198$, $P < 0.001$). At three months, in terms of the effects in change in clinical practice, overall, 24 per cent of attendees had used a problem focused clinical assessment in the last week and 40 per cent of attendees reported using one or more CBSH workbooks per week (Williams *et al.*, 2010). Interventions that we have offered to help improve this and maintain application in practice include local monthly Five Areas discussion groups led by local 'leads'/trainers or other advocates of the approach, such as a local 'champion'.

Overcoming three common problems during training

Q One person dominates by asking/answering all the questions

Possible response

'It's great you've so many ideas from the training. We're keen also to hear from others on the course as well. Does anyone else have any other ideas?'

Alternative responses

- Ask general/open questions to which there aren't 'right' answers.
- Use small groups: Get people talking and answering questions in small groups, and rotate the groups so the more vocal person doesn't come to work with (and dominate) the same two to three people each time.
- Use the 'teaching rules' that were jointly agreed in the very first training session. These should be planned from the start to include the opportunity for all to take part/contribute. This can be gently pointed to e.g. 'Thanks for that Lisa, you're quite right, but now I want to also help everyone else get their comments in as well so that we make sure we meet our training goal from session 1, that everyone can get the chance to contribute.'

- Steps on from there might be to try jokes, e.g. 'Lisa, you're going to wear yourself out! Just for the moment I'm going to ask you to hold back to give everyone a chance.'
- The next step would be to talk privately before or after a session and ask for a change in behaviour ('It's really great how much you contribute – but we need to give others the chance. We want you to keep contributing by being here, but we have to ask that you limit the amount you respond to just three times today').

No-one answers/everyone sits silently looking at the floor

Possible response

Split the larger class up into smaller discussion groups of two to three people. Then fuse the small groups into a larger group and ask them to share/summarise what they have talked about. Set it up so the same person doesn't summarise both times.

Someone is rude and dismissive

Possible response

Remind everyone of the training rules, and the need to have a good atmosphere for training. If the person continues to be rude, or has come intoxicated or disturbed, you could call for a coffee break and speak to them quietly and ask them to leave for this week.

If the same person continues to cause problems, you could take them on one side before a future training session to give a last warning, and ultimately ask them to leave the class. For practitioner groups this situation is very unlikely; however if you believe someone is suffering from alcohol or drug dependency then referring them to their manager and considering a formal report to their professional body is appropriate.

Training in the Five Areas approach

Several different training courses are available for using the Five Areas approach. These vary from half a day to four-day courses.

Short introduction sessions (one to three hours)

- Overview of the Five Areas approach.
- Introducing and supporting the Five Areas resources.

One-day courses

- Using the Five Areas approach in community settings.
- Overcoming depression and low mood (book).
- Using the Living Life to the Full (LLTTF) books, DVD and online course.
- Using the Living Life to the Full Interactive online course.
- Five Areas approach to eating disorders.
- Using the LLTTF classes.

Two-day course

- LLTTF classes.

Three-day courses

SPIRIT (using *Overcoming depression and low mood* and *Overcoming anxiety, stress and panic*). SPIRIT stands for Structured Psychosocial InteRventions in Teams.

Evaluating the training courses

The main Five Areas training (SPIRIT) disk contains a number of handouts and evaluation forms that helps record baseline, during and end evaluations of learning. This examines self-rated knowledge and skills gains as well as objective measures of learning gains.

Research in the training courses

Research examining two of the training courses has been published:

- Ahmed S, Joice A, Kent C, Williams CJ. (2007) Introducing CBT self-help approaches into condition management teams. *Mental Health and Learning Disabilities Research and Practice* **4**(2): 175–188. Available as a free download from **www.fiveareas.com**.
- Williams C, Dafters R, Ronald L, Martinez R, Garland A. (2010) Training practitioners in cognitive behavioural self-help – the SPIRIT (Structured Psychosocial InteRventions in Teams) Project. *Behavioural and Cognitive Psychotherapy.*

We would welcome hearing about any other local evaluations that have been done elsewhere.

Online training resources

Several websites contain useful information for practitioners:

1) **www.fiveareas.com** – providing access to the whole range of Five Areas resources, including free downloads.
2) **www.fiveareastraining.com** has a range of online modules addressing the Five Areas course.
3) **www.livinglifetothefull.com** (short-cut **www.llttf.com**) has all the key modules you need to get going and use the popular Living Life to the Full course. It includes practitioner training resources on the Plan, Do, Review model and a Quick start guide to using the course.

Arranging training

It is possible to arrange training days (one to three day courses) to be delivered at a local training event by the Five Areas training team. A number of trainers who are located around the UK can provide sessions to your service. To arrange this, please contact training@fiveareas.com. We can also provide a 'training the trainers' CD-Rom of training resources so that training can be delivered on site by local trainers and champions for sustainability (see below).

Key practice points

- It matters more to be comprehensible than to be comprehensive. In other words, teaching key points that are clearly communicated, and that can be learned and applied is what is needed. The rule 'Teach people less and they will remember more' is often true.

Support resources

Online resources

Free to download from **www.fiveareas.com**:

- Planner sheet.
- Review sheet.

Practitioner training: **www.fiveareastraining.com**.

Train the trainer resources

Training courses for Five Areas training are available for use under licence. They contain the licensed resources listed in Box 11.2

Needing more help?

A range of training support and advice is available. Please contact training@fiveareas.com for information about local training and resources.

Box 11.2 Five Areas training resources (available under licence as a training disk from **www.fiveareas.com**)

1. **One-day workshop and handout:**
   - Making the Five Areas approach work for you and your service (PowerPoint file).
   - Handout (Making the Five Areas approach work for you and your service).
2. **Short session modules** (based on (1) above and aimed at shorter presentations).
3. **Large CBT Books course** (addressing *Overcoming depression and low mood* and key elements of *Overcoming anxiety, stress and panic*). Sessions covered are:
   - Introduction/overview to the course.
   - Clinical assessment.
   - Introducing and using CBT self-help.
   - Reduced activity, avoidance, and building exercise.
   - Noticing and changing extreme and unhelpful thinking.
   - Practical problem solving, helpful and unhelpful behaviours
   - Assertiveness, irritability, communication, building relationships, information for families and friends.
   - Medication, improving sleep and healthy living.
   - Planning for the future and after the course.
4. **Key resource handouts:**
   - Planner and Review sheets.
   - Overview sheets: Using the Little CBT Books.
   - Quick-start guides to various Five Areas resources.

References

Blackburn IM, James IA, Milne DL, Baker C, Standart S, Garland A, Reichelt FK. (2001) The revised cognitive therapy scale (CTS-R): psychometric properties. *Behavioural and Cognitive Psychotherapy* **29**: 431–46.

Keeley H, Williams CJ, Shapiro D. (2002) A United Kingdom survey of accredited cognitive behaviour therapists' attitudes towards and use of structured self-help materials. *Behavioural and Cognitive Psychotherapy* **30**: 191–201.

Layard R. (2006) The case for psychological treatment centres. *BMJ* **332**: 1030–2.

National Institute for Health and Clinical Excellence (NICE). (2007) *Anxiety: Management of anxiety in adults in primary, secondary and community settings*. Clinical guideline 22. London: National Institute for Health and Clinical Excellence.

National Institute for Health and Clinical Excellence (NICE). (2009) *Depression: Management of depression in primary and secondary care*. Clinical guideline 90. London: National Institute for Health and Clinical Excellence.

Scottish Intercollegiate Guidelines Network (SIGN). (2010) Guideline 114: *Non-pharmaceutical treatment of depression in adults: A national clinical guideline*. Available at: **www.sign.ac.uk/pdf/sign114.pdf**.

Skills for Health. (2008a) See **http://www.ucl.ac.uk/clinical-psychology/CORE/CBT_Framework.htm**.

Skills for Health. (2008b) **See https://tools.skillsforhealth.org.uk/suite/show/id/81**.

Whitfield G, Williams CJ. (2004) If the evidence is so good why doesn't anyone use them? Current uses of computer-based self-help packages. *Behavioural and Cognitive Psychotherapy* **32**: 57–65.

Williams C. (2009) Guided CBT Rating Scale. Available at: **www.fiveareas.com**.

Williams C, Dafters R, Ronald L, Martinez R, Garland A. (2010) Training the wider workforce in cognitive behavioural self-help \ndash; the SPIRIT (Structured Psychosocial InteRventions in Teams) Training course. *Behavioural and Cognitive Psychotherapy.*

Further reading

Keeley H, Williams CJ, Shapiro D. (2002) A United Kingdom survey of accredited cognitive behaviour therapists' attitudes towards and use of structured self-help materials. *Behavioural and Cognitive Psychotherapy* **30**: 191–201.

Scottish Intercollegiate Guidelines Network (SIGN). (2010) Guideline 114: *Non-pharmaceutical treatment of depression in adults: A national clinical guideline*. Available at: **www.sign.ac.uk/pdf/sign114.pdf**.

Whitfield G, Williams CJ. (2004) If the evidence is so good why doesn't anyone use them? Current uses of computer-based self-help packages. *Behavioural and Cognitive Psychotherapy* **32**: 57–65.

PART 5

The Five Areas in action

Introduction

The Five Areas model is already being applied in several countries across a range of settings and in a variety of disorders. This section of the book aims to a illustrate a small part of the experience that has been gained by different services with these new ways of working. This includes the challenges faced by different practitioners while supporting people and success stories that they are proud of and want to share. Central to each project has been the idea of working differently and providing something that combines an approach that is evidence based and is attractive to practitioners and users alike.

Several things stand out:

- The Five Areas model provides in itself a way of making sense of things that helps practitioners then offer a range of linked interventions, which can include guided CBT, and more. In other words the Five Areas assessment can be de-coupled from the use of the self-help resources and is valuable as a tool in its own right.
- Delivery within the health service ranges from general practice attendees and Increasing Access to Psychological Therapies (IAPT)-style teams through to staff working with patients with complex long-term problems attending tertiary specialist clinics.
- Many of the interventions are focused outside the health service, with delivery in schools by teachers and educational psychologists, by housing workers, by social services, as well as by staff and volunteers working in the voluntary sector.
- Establishing a new service can take time and requires adjustment and constant problem solving.
- Delivery can include face to face working, telephone support, email and group classes.
- The Living Life to the Full (LLTTF) classes have proved popular among adults, older adults and young people.
- Online approaches can be attractive as a first step to care and may work best with people who have their own access to the internet. It provides access to an evidence-based approach that has the potential to engage people who have not received support before.
- A wide range of access is possible – both within and also from outside the health service – with direct referral providing a new and important way of helping people access help.

While reading this chapter, practitioners should consider aspects that transfer well to their patients, and work in their setting. Remember also the statement by the German General von Moltke that 'no battle plan survives contact with the enemy'. In other words, the plans within which practitioners monitor and seek feedback should be adjustable and modified as needed to meet the needs of each individual patient. This flexibility comes through loud and clear in a number of the descriptions that follow and explains much of their success.

Five Areas model as a first contact assessment tool in an IAPT team in England

Practitioners	Samantha Cox, Mark Hudson, Sarah Benson, Tracy Wright, trainee psychological wellbeing practitioners, based in Derbyshire, UK
Setting	Right Steps Turning Point Service, Amber Valley and Erewash
Population	General practice patients: 4500, age 16 +, experiencing low mood/anxiety
Five Areas intervention(s) being delivered	We use the Five Areas model as a formulation tool in assessment to identify the main problem statement and to aid understanding by the patient, so they can see how their symptoms interrelate and are maintaining their problem. We also use Five Areas to help guide our low intensity interventions. A large amount of our support is delivered over the telephone.
How did you match what was offered to meet the person's needs?	The introductory call informs us of any accessibility issues, which will include literacy or language barriers. Following on from this at the assessment, the client will be asked what they hope to achieve from treatment. This helps us in choosing appropriate material to match their needs and requirements. We offer a range of resources to meet this; these include the (Little CBT) Books, (Big Book) workbooks, DVD, cCBT and self-help classes.
Who is supporting/ delivering this work?	IAPT workers in conjunction with others involved in patients care.
How did you introduce the approach?	By follow-up telephone calls after the assessment and case management supervision.
What has gone well?	It formulates people's problems in a structured and focused way that is easy to understand by them also over the telephone. As an example, we have had several clients who have found the DVD helpful in realising they are not alone in their problems, and in informing them more about their problem. Another client has found the *Overcoming Anxiety* book really useful in identifying and challenging unhelpful thoughts that are maintaining their anxiety.
What hasn't gone so well?	Not always easy to explain over the telephone within a telephone service. Not always easy to fit client's problem within a Five Areas model. Sometimes clients find it difficult to think of specific situation that relates well to their problem. It is harder to do if there are co-morbidity problems, particularly within the time-frame.
What problems were there, and how have you worked to overcome any problems?	By asking the client what they see as their main difficulty if there is co-morbidity and focusing on this as their specific example. Asking clients what physical symptoms they experience first starts the thought process about the Five Areas.
What have you learned from working in this way?	It provides a good, clear structure for the assessment. It is simple to understand and the vicious circle provides a clear rationale for maintenance and informing treatment.
What's been the overall impact?	Too early to say because we are beginning to start treatments and will not know until the treatment is complete. We have been able, however, to make contact and carry out several hundred assessments within a short space of time.
What is the single greatest benefit?	Simplicity and jargon-free language.

→

Any hints and tips for others?	Involving the patient is vital and ask them which areas they want to work on and what they see as being the benefits of treatment. Make it idiosyncratic so that they really engage.
Further details	Samantha Cox, Mark Hudson, Sarah Benson, Tracy Wright, Turning Point, Unity Mill House, Derwent Street, Belper, Derbyshire DE56 1WN, UK. Tel: 01773 596201; **www.turning-point.co.uk** Rightsteps Working together for wellbeing and recovery

Five Areas books with GP support

Name	Dr Stephen Williams, GP partner
Setting	UK-based general practice/community setting in a village/town setting
Population	General practice patients
Five Areas intervention being delivered	The Five Areas model is used within the practice primarily for patients presenting with depression and anxiety with a particular emphasis on those with co-morbid physical medical conditions. The goals of introducing the approach into a GP setting include: • Enhancing the treatment of common mental health problems. • Avoiding inappropriate use of pharmacological treatment particularly for moderate and mild presentations. • Increasing patient choice. • Improving patient self-efficacy and reducing inappropriate clinician dependence. • Improving the management of long-term medical conditions (e.g. diabetes, chronic obstructive pulmonary disease (COPD), ischaemic heart disease) with associated co-morbid depression and anxiety thereby improving outcomes and reducing costs. • Providing primary care clinicians with basic CBT-based skills. • Encouraging a psychosocial approach within the practice that encourages 'psychological mindedness' for both patients and clinicians.
How did you match what was offered to meet the person's needs?	Primarily provision of written materials based on the Five Areas model both unsupported within a self-help area and offered/'prescribed' by clinicians. Patients were previously offered the CD-Rom version of the Five Areas model but this had a relatively low take-up when delivered in an open waiting area setting at the practice. Patients are currently frequently referred to the Livinglifetothefull.com website as an alternative that avoids the need for use of printed materials etc.
Who is supporting/ delivering this work?	For example, GP partners, practice nurses, voluntary workers. Five Areas self-help materials are used by other GP partners to a limited extent and by practice nurses. The most successful usage has been by nurse practitioners, who have developed a relatively high degree of expertise in using the approach. I (SMW) provide back-up and 'consultancy' in the form of additional longer (30-minute) sessions within the practice where supported self-help in isolation appears insufficient. I also provide 'supervision' to other team members, particularly nurse practitioners.

How did you introduce the approach?	The initial step was to involve and 'sell' the benefits of the Five Areas approach to the whole practice team. The practice had a pre-existing self-help room into which the Five Areas materials were introduced. Simultaneously, a limited number of practice members attended 'Five Areas' workshops and I undertook some training of other team members myself.
What has gone well?	The use of written self-help materials based on the Five Areas approach has been the single most effective intervention, based on patient and clinician feedback. As noted, nurse practitioners continue to use the approach most consistently. A system of referral to myself for patients requiring more than brief Five Areas interventions has generally worked well.
What hasn't gone so well?	Usage by GPs partners and practice nurses has been more erratic. The use of a CD version of the Five Areas approach was not successful in practice when it was delivered in a large shared room.
What problems were there, and how have you worked to overcome any problems?	Initial concerns about the cost of printing self-help materials were overcome by involving the surgery patient support group. This is also now less important with increasing use of downloadable patient materials via the 'Living life to the full' website. The greatest single problem has been in maintaining my role as providing support and supervision for other clinicians using the approach, rather than being used as a referral service.
What have you learned from working in this way?	At a personal level the importance of providing a role which supports active patient use of self-help materials rather than being in the role of a 'therapist'. This in turn 'resonates' with the difficulties in providing support and supervision to other team members whilst resisting the temptation to too easily adopt the role of a referral agency.
What's been the overall impact?	The practice has long regarded itself as relatively 'psychologically minded' and adopting the Five Areas model does appear to have helped to maintain this approach, particularly in the face of additional external pressures. This in turn helps to maintain low rates of referrals to primary and secondary care including an emphasis on avoiding inappropriate referrals of patients with medically unexplained symptoms.
What is the single greatest benefit?	The Five Areas model potentially provides an additional 'level' of intervention, which when working well achieves effective and supportive therapeutic collaboration between patients and clinicians.
Any hints and tips for others?	The importance of early involvement of the whole primary care team as far as possible. Delegating responsibility for practical tasks such as maintenance of written materials to a dedicated (administrative) team member. Continuing emphasis on communication, supervision, and discussion of difficulties and feedback of successes.
Any other comments?	None, other than the increased sense of 'self-efficacy', which can result from this approach for both patients and clinicians.

Five Areas depression book plus telephone support in Canada

Practitioner	Mark Lau, clinical psychologist, Vancouver, British Columbia (BC), Canada
Setting	Telephone support is provided by 20 coaches located in Canadian Mental Health Association-BC Division branch offices in 17 urban and rural communities in BC.
Population	Primary care patients aged 19 or older experiencing mild to moderate depression with or without anxiety. As of June 2010, approximately 7000 referrals had been made to the programme.
Five Areas intervention being delivered	Bounce Back: Reclaim your health (BB) provides telephone support to primary care patients with mild to moderate depression in their use of the *Overcoming depression, low mood and anxiety: a Five Areas approach** (OD) self-help materials. This programme was developed to bridge the gap between the need for mental health services by these patients and the lack of availability of these services in BC. The content of the self-help materials (including psycho-educational DVD and self-help mood improvement workbook) was adapted for a BC context. Telephone support is provided over three to five sessions for a total contact time of approximately two to two and half hours.
How did you match what was offered to meet the person's needs?	Bounce Back offers two forms of help. The first is a 45-minute DVD providing practical tips on managing mood and healthy living. This DVD is a good, first-line intervention for individuals who could benefit from learning about self-help strategies but don't like to use workbooks. The second Bounce Back resource offers support to patients by a community-based coach in the use of the OD workbook. In order to best meet the needs of BC primary care patients, this new mental health service is delivered to patients via telephone in their own homes and patients' use of the OD self-help materials is supported via trained coaches.
Who is supporting/ delivering this work?	Telephone support is provided by community-based non-specialist coaches who were hired and trained specifically to support the use of the OD materials over the telephone. The coaches participated in a three-day training workshop in how to provide support for the OD self-help materials. This training was followed by weekly telephone consultations with a clinical psychologist to reinforce knowledge and skill development, to provide clinical support, and to reinforce the focus on the self-help materials. As the coaches have become more experienced, telephone consultations have been tapered to once a month.
How did you introduce the approach?	The Bounce Back programme was introduced to the general practitioners by the coaches.
What has gone well?	The programme has fulfilled its promise by leading to improvements in self-reported mood and anxiety symptoms, physical health and quality of life for primary care patients with mild to moderate levels of depression. The programme has been well received by primary care physicians. The decisions to provide support by telephone has made participation more convenient for patients and improved the reach of the programme. Finally, the training of the non-specialist coaches was effective and resulted in the coaches delivering the programme with good fidelity.

→

What hasn't gone so well?	It took some time for primary care physicians and other stakeholders to see the Bounce Back programme as a credible and ongoing community-based support. One consequence of using the telephone is that patients may be more likely to miss scheduled appointments.
What problems were there, and how have you worked to overcome any problems?	First, in order to ensure that the programme was delivered in an equitable fashion across the province, clear policies and procedures were developed. Second, the non-specialist coaches came with a range of previous clinical experiences. The solution was to develop an effective training programme comprised of a three-day workshop and weekly group telephone consultations to ensure that all coaches provided telephone support in a similar fashion.
What have you learned from working in this way?	The success of this programme has taught us that it is possible to deliver a low intensity/high capacity intervention to primary care patients. Non-specialist coaches can be effective in supporting CBT self-help. Community-based organisations can partner with the healthcare system. From an operational perspective, implementing the programme on a community by community basis has not proved as efficient as a regional model.
What's been the overall impact?	An independent interim qualitative evaluation reports full implementation, with sound clinical quality assurance, monitoring and risk management processes, of the BB programme has been achieved. There is also growing support from primary care for the program and BB is perceived by stakeholders as a credible and valued intervention. A quantitative evaluation of the first 600 BB patients who completed the OD self-help programme with telephone coaching demonstrates a positive impact of the programme on self-reported mood and anxiety symptoms, physical health and quality of life.
What is the single greatest benefit?	Bounce Back is the first programme of its kind in BC. It has been able to help many primary care patients with mild to moderate depression who otherwise would not have received mental health services.
Any hints and tips for others?	Implementing a province-wide programme requires a dedicated team. In addition, centralised clinical oversight has ensured equitable delivery of the programme across the province.
Further details	**www.cmha.bc.ca/bounceback** BounceBack reclaim your health British Columbia The Best Place on Earth — Ministry of Health Services
Any other comments?	*This book is a version of the *Overcoming depression and low mood book*, which has been especially printed for the project and includes additional workbooks from *Overcoming anxiety*, so the book combines low mood, worry, panic and tackling avoidance as well as the wider range of interventions for depression.

Use of the *Overcoming anxiety* book in an IAPT service

Practitioner	Emma Nutting, psychological wellbeing practitioner
Setting	Lincolnshire Partnership NHS Foundation Trust (Psychological Therapies and Primary Care)
Population	Adults of working age experiencing mild to moderate common mental health problems
Five Areas intervention being delivered	*Overcoming anxiety: a Five Areas approach* (Individual workbooks)
How did you match what was offered to meet the person's needs?	Psychological wellbeing practitioners offer assessment to clients who have been identified via their GP or a triage nurse to be suffering from a mild to moderate common mental health problem. Through this assessment the psychological wellbeing practitioners in conjunction with the client agree on what intervention will be offered.
Who is supporting/ delivering this work?	Psychological wellbeing practitioners.
How did you introduce the approach?	Psychological wellbeing practitioners present the approach to clients in a 1:1 face to face contact. The Five Areas model is introduced to the client and completed using a recent example of when they felt anxious. Following this the most relevant part of the model is identified (e.g. thoughts, feelings, symptoms, behaviours or practical problems) and the client is given a workbook related to this.
What has gone well?	Clients report that the materials are clear, concise, and easy to understand and like the fact that the workbooks take them through a step-by-step process. Clients also state that they like that the workbooks offer examples and then provide space for clients to write down their own examples. This creates great opportunity to start to understand why they feel as they do whilst giving something to relate to. In addition to this clients can work through the workbooks in their own time and at their own pace. As clients can be followed up and supported either through face to face contact or telephone contact, it creates greater flexibility.
What hasn't gone so well?	Some clients find it difficult to engage to work in a guided self-help way. Therefore it was important to state from the outset what is expected from both parties. In this instance it became important to be positive about the approach and sell its benefits.
What problems were there, and how have you worked to overcome any problems?	Some clients either forgot to bring their workbooks with them or lost them completely. Psychological wellbeing practitioners found that it was important to have spare materials to hand or send additional copies out to clients.
What have you learned from working in this way?	Clients enjoy being empowered and to feel that they are solving their own problems. The skills are transferable; therefore once clients understand the approach they are able to adapt the skills to new situations as they arise. Sometimes just by supporting someone to understand the interaction between thoughts, feelings and activity can be enough to help them feel better.

→

What's been the overall impact?	• Increased awareness of what anxiety is and its causes. • Reduced anxiety and low mood. • An understanding of the relationship between thoughts, feelings and activity. • Increased self-confidence and self-esteem. • Increased activity and a reduction in avoidant behaviour. • Reduction in negative thoughts. • Increased sense of control. • Increased wellbeing. • A sense of empowerment.
What is the single greatest benefit?	It allows clients to learn how to help themselves.
Any hints and tips for others?	Ensure that you fully understand the model. Keep your resources well stocked and be flexible with your clients. Ensure that clients understand the importance of the homework element of guided self-help.
Further details	Emma Nutting, psychological wellbeing practitioner Emma.Nutting@LPFT.nhs.uk
Any other comments?	The resources are very user-friendly for clients and clinicians.

Little CBT Books delivered by housing workers in England

Practitioner	Leon Herbert, Safe Inside, Safe Outside (SISO), project manager and housing support practitioner, Leicester, UK
Setting	City in the UK
Population	Mental health service users – 8000, age 18–65, experiencing low mood/anxiety
Five Areas intervention being delivered	The SISO Team made up of mental health service users have used the 'Little Booklets' series as a self-help peer support section of the *SISO for wellbeing toolkit*. The SISO team are also currently delivering workshops across the East Midlands and South East to other mental health service users and mental health support staff and services, who will all receive a *SISO for Wellbeing Toolkit* and an overview of how to use/get the best out of the little booklets allied to the information on the Five Areas/CBT overview and national IAPT programme picture for service users and mental health support managers and staff to use and incorporate into their lives/practice.
How did you match what was offered to meet the person's needs?	By giving a comprehensive overview and context of IAPT/CBT and Five Areas allied to a full range of Little Booklets and self-help guide (contained in the 'Techniques for raising energies and lifting spirits' section of the *SISO for wellbeing toolkit*. Also contains signposting links to Five Areas websites and materials.
Who is supporting/ delivering this work?	Mental health service users in a peer support capacity, and mental health practitioners and support workers via the *SISO for wellbeing toolkit*.

→

How did you introduce the approach?	By putting the national picture into context, the resources and guidance were identified by the SISO team of mental health service users as an important tool and component in their own recovery journey via the two-year Department of Health funded Recovery-In-Action Programme. SISO is now moving towards the creation of its own Social Enterprise.
What has gone well?	The adaptability of the Five Areas resources as self-help tools and subsequent website materials – helping to break the cycle of unhelpful thinking and ensuring everyone from service users to staff understand the national context of IAPT and CBT, with the Five Areas and associated materials acting as a conduit to this. Overall it is assisting people to reclaim their lives and make the recovery journey a reality by making long-standing problems manageable.
What hasn't gone so well?	Occasionally we have had some resistance from 'longstanding professionals' who are entrenched in a different era of practice; trying to open their minds up has on occasions been challenging.
What problems were there, and how have you worked to overcome any problems?	See above. By giving taster exercises and hearing from service users the help it has given them in their own recovery journey. Encouraging them to read the section around IAPT/CBT and Five Areas, always being accessible to offer support and guidance to any questions given.
What have you learned from working in this way?	That it is empowering and offers real solutions in a self-management style and non-clinical language, which real people understand and relate to. It offers quick and meaningful solutions for long-standing problems and issues for people.
What's been the overall impact?	Prevention of small problems becoming oversized and unmanageable. It also makes prevention in a more general sense a real possibility as it breaks that painful cycle of unhelpful thinking.
What is the single greatest benefit?	Empowerment, self-management and a genuine understanding of how and why we think and process information in the way that we do. It really assists people in getting to know themselves better and gives recognition and solutions to the problems or inequalities in their lives which continues to hold them back.
Any hints and tips for others?	The Five Areas work really allows people to examine and break down a problem or difficulty in a panoramic way that ensures that problems which affect life and behaviour are manageable and can be a small part of life rather than the very definition of who you are as a person.
Further details	Leon Herbert, SISO project manager, Advance Support, 5 Faraday Court, Conduit Street, Leicester LE2 0JN, UK; tel: 0116 2553200; **www.advanceuk.org**; **www.advancesupport.org** (look for the SISO link); **www.refugemusic.co.uk**
Any other comments?	Only that this work will go from strength to strength and assist many others in becoming more independent and in control of the issues that continue to hold them back, regardless of what situation or background you are from.

Little CBT Books delivered by social services via telephone and LLTTF classes

Practitioner	Young Foundation, centre for social innovation based in London, UK
Setting	Based in South Tyneside in community settings
Population	People aged 65 and over who are suffering from mild depression or anxiety, social isolation, financial exclusion, ill health or bereavement.
Five Areas intervention being delivered	We are piloting the course of 'Little CBT Books' (named 'Full of Life' for this pilot) for people aged 65 and over as both individual telephone support and group sessions.
How did you match what was offered to meet the person's needs?	The telephone support was a model that could be adapted to meet each individual's needs. The volunteers and the service users had an initial conversation to discuss their reasons for wanting support and to choose three or four out of the seven booklets that they felt were most relevant to them. The volunteers and the service users then arranged the phone calls for a time that suited them. The service users could ask for anything between one and five sessions. The group sessions covered all of the booklets as a series but sessions could focus on particular aspects that the group felt they could gain most from.
Who is supporting/ delivering this work?	The Full of Life course is being delivered by trained local volunteers of the same age range. The pilot is being managed by members of the Adult Duty Team and Adult Social Services team at South Tyneside Metropolitan Borough Council, and the Young Foundation. The council set up a steering group in the early stages of the pilot, which consists of local third sector organisations and the primary care trust. Through promotional activities they have also secured the buy-in of district nurses and residential care homes.
How did you introduce the approach?	Full of Life was introduced to local authority staff as an effective – and cost-effective – way of improving the wellbeing of the growing number of older people in the area. Until recently initiatives to increase the wellbeing of older people have tended to focus on physical and health needs. Comparatively little focus has been placed on mental health issues such as depression, which have relatively high prevalence in later life. Full of Life was introduced as a service to fill this gap. The life skills that can be learnt from CBT-based approaches can help people of all ages to cope better with challenges and transitions. We highlighted that Full of Life was a service that would create a 'win–win' situation, in which the wellbeing of the clients would increase through using the service and the wellbeing of the volunteers would improve through delivering the service, remaining active in the community and re-engaging with their professional skills.
What has gone well?	• Training: The volunteers have been enthusiastic about the training they received from Dr Chris Williams and his team and they felt confident in their understanding of the materials and how to guide others through them. • Delivery: Initial feedback from older people who have gone through the telephone support has been positive. They found the booklets accessible, easy to use, helpful, and relevant to their day-to-day lives and issues. All of them enjoyed their interactions with the volunteers they had been assigned to.

→

What hasn't gone so well?	Recruiting clients onto the course has been slow. There is a clear need for this type of service, but local authority staff perhaps focused too much at the beginning of this project on promoting the service as only a mental health service, rather than a more holistic service that teaches and reinforces everyday life skills that can support people through difficult situations and transitions. We have subsequently worked closely with the team to ensure promotion of the course highlights the 'Full of Life' concept more fully.
What problems were there, and how have you worked to overcome any problems?	As above, initially there was a low take-up from older people in the area; it became clear quite quickly that more time was needed talking with potential service users to ensure that they had an adequate understanding of what the books were like and how they would be supported to use them. Project staff were also trained to ensure they promoted Full of Life not just as a mental health service. Promotional materials have been produced and distributed; an 'awareness raising day' was held for agencies that work with older people in South Tyneside; and project staff have visited care homes in person to talk through the booklets.
What have you learned from working in this way?	We have learnt that local council can work successfully with local community members and the voluntary sector and that Full of Life is complementary to the existing local authority befriending services and mental health initiatives; that volunteers can be trained to guide older people through materials confidently; and that this model of working has a positive impact on both volunteers and clients.
What's been the overall impact?	Full of Life has increased the wellbeing of the client group as well as those who volunteered to facilitate the materials.
What is the single greatest benefit?	Improving the wellbeing of the local older population.
Any hints and tips for others?	Ensure that all team members fully understand the materials and what the course is aiming to tackle – ensure that all staff involved with this course attend at least the first day of training even if they are not delivering the materials, as this helped with the promotion of the service to clients.
Further details	**www.youngfoundation.org** THE YOUNG FOUNDATION

LLTTF classes delivered in community settings

Practitioner	Pat Lynch, Aware Defeat Depression charity
Setting	Community settings in several areas of Northern Ireland
Population	Adults affected by mild/moderate depression/anxiety
Five Areas intervention being delivered	Living Life To The Full classes
How did you match what was offered to meet the person's needs?	The classes were delivered to groups of 10–14 people and so difficult to meet everyone's needs. In the publicity literature we gave details of content and who the course was suitable for. At the commencement of each course we spent some time discussing participants' expectations and tried to ensure that these were met.
Who is supporting/ delivering this work?	The work is partially funded by the DHSS & PS Northern Ireland and individual health trusts. It is delivered by a number of facilitators who meet selection criteria specified by our CBT expert, who is a cognitive therapy trainer. Facilitators typically have experience of working with people with mental health problems, training experience, group work skills and good knowledge of CBT.
How did you introduce the approach?	It is being piloted at several locations at present and participants self-refer or are being referred by GPs, mental health professionals. All participants are given information about the programme and encouraged to attend all sessions. Further information is given at the initial session.
What has gone well?	Participants in general rate the social aspect of the programme very highly and the evaluations to date have been very favourable. We have an external evaluator and use GHQ12s before and after. To date the vast majority of attendees have shown significant improvement in GHQ scores following completion of the course. Participants also relate well to most of the materials and activities and are impressed by the high standard of resources.
What hasn't gone so well?	Not that much really so far. There will always be some people for whom the course is not suitable. It can also be difficult at times to pitch it at the right level for a range of people and to ensure that one or more people do not dominate in discussions.
What problems were there, and how have you worked to overcome any problems?	Finding an ideal venue in terms of room size/ambience/accessibility can be difficult – so we have worked hard at this. Also the need for high social element has become apparent in feedback so have left time for tea/coffee/chat. Also experimenting with evening/daytime courses and with number of sessions as it is a bit of a balancing act – the more sessions the more likely you are to lose people along the way. We try to make the classes as enjoyable as possible for participants on the basis that if people enjoy something they will learn and will also come back. The other main problem is making GPs aware of the courses and getting them to refer patients. We are still working on this.

→

What have you learned from working in this way?	We have learned that most people enjoy interaction with other human beings although initially many people can be very apprehensive. So it is important to make everyone feel welcome and to encourage a bond between group members. We notice that after a few sessions most people are much more relaxed. It is also essential to pick up on any warning signs and in this regard we always have two facilitators in case someone becomes upset. Inevitably there may be a small amount of personal disclosure but we keep this to a minimum.
What's been the overall impact?	So far it has been very significant – we know this from informal feedback and from GHQ12s.
What is the single greatest benefit?	The most significant benefit is that a group of people can have access to a high-quality educational programme based on CBT concepts and it appears to date that for many people this is sufficient to motivate them to help themselves make significant changes in their lifestyle and challenge negative and extreme thinking patterns.
Any hints and tips for others?	Probably said it all before but I suppose the main thing would be for facilitators/trainers to use the resources as a framework to deliver the course – don't let the resources use you. Observe the group and get a feel if something is or isn't working – don't be afraid to break people into groups or pairs and in general the more participative the classes are the better. It is important to help individuals with some of the activities – get among them as some people need encouragement or perhaps more information to complete some of the sheets. Also have good information about local resources that people can access during and after the course.
Further details	www.aware-ni.org
Any other comments?	aware DEFEAT DEPRESSION

DHSS & PS, Department of Health, Social Services and Public Safety.

LLTTF classes with university students

Practitioner	Kirsten Thomlinson, low intensity practitioner, Depression Alliance Scotland (DAS), UK
Setting	Various community settings, Edinburgh, Scotland, UK
Population	We recruited 17 people onto the course, with one two-hour session each week over an eight-week period. We held a follow-up session six weeks after the final session.
Five Areas intervention being delivered	An eight-week LLTTF course to students at Edinburgh University. The course focuses on strategies to help students manage mood and deal with common problems associated with low mood and depression. The intervention is set within our campaign, Look OK ... Feel Crap? (**www.lookokfeelcrap.org**), and aims to increase knowledge of depression among young adults in Scotland and encourage more young people to seek help. We approached Edinburgh University Counselling Service as partners in this intervention to target students specifically. Depression, low mood and anxiety consistently make up a large proportion of those seeking counselling support. The goal with this intervention is to offer students practical self-help support, based on a CBT approach, in a non-stigmatising setting.
How did you match what was offered to meet the person's needs?	The course includes a mixture of presentation, group discussion and individual work and is backed-up by a range of resources to aid learning. All students received weekly course handouts, Five Areas booklets and a CBT workbook. The course structure is flexible so we could shape discussion towards topics that students themselves had identified as areas of concern. Staff were on hand during the session and by email over the week to answer any specific questions that people may have.
Who is delivering this work?	The intervention was delivered by two course leaders: a Depression Alliance Scotland community development officer alongside a counsellor from Edinburgh University Counselling Service.
How did you introduce the approach?	We have delivered two courses at Edinburgh University. The first course was advertised on the student union portal as an open-referral course. The second course was through referral from both the Edinburgh University Counselling Service and the Health Service. The courses were delivered on campus to make it easier for students to attend the weekly sessions and also to minimise the stigma commonly associated with accessing mental health services.
What has gone well?	Over the duration of the course, the students developed into a very supportive unit. They were increasingly willing to share personal thoughts with others. A notable success was the decision by the students to continue to meet informally after the course had finished in support of each other. This is a superb example of individual students taking the initiative to put what they had learned in action.
What hasn't gone so well?	The preparation for each session required more planning with the partnership approach. Planning meetings had to be scheduled into both trainers' diaries and sufficient time had to be set aside for debriefing sessions. The DAS worker was lead trainer for the course and supported the counselling staff member in participating in delivery as the course progressed.

→

What problems were there, and how have you worked to overcome any problems?	Encouraging students to speak in front of the large group was a challenge. Students identified perfectionism as one area of concern, and there was certainly reluctance to voice comments or thoughts in front of others. We overcame this by increasing the time spent doing small group work, inviting students to form into groups of two to three people to complete work tasks. Another problem was ensuring people understand that what works for one person might not work for everyone. For example, some well-meaning participants think everyone should complete the thought programme in a certain way, which caused others to feel pressured into doing something that they didn't find helpful. Talking this over as a group resolved any stress.
What have you learned from working in this way?	The partnership approach has worked particularly well. Inviting Edinburgh University Counselling service to co-deliver the course with us brought a much-welcome 'insider' perspective to group discussion. Our aim in working in this way was to give staff working inside the service the skills necessary either to deliver the course themselves or to use the approach in one-to-one sessions. This enables us to then move on and work with new organisations and over time increase the numbers of young adults we can reach.
What's been the overall impact?	The analysis showed that the students had increased in their knowledge and understanding of low mood and improved their ability in tackling common problems. They rated the group discussion as the most helpful activity. This is in contrast to their reluctance to talk at the beginning of the course, but shows the impact that sharing has on people, once trust has been established among group members. Individual and small group work was also rated highly. The Five Areas diagram was rated as the most helpful learning in the course, giving people something practical to work with and use in their own lives. Relaxation skills (anxiety control training), assertiveness skills and dealing with unhelpful thoughts were also rated highly.
What is the single greatest benefit?	Having a well-evidenced course appropriate for use in community settings and with high-quality resources is of huge benefit to us. The flexibility of Five Areas means we have used it many different organisations, with similarly positive results.
Any hints and tips for others?	Gathering evaluation data is always a challenge. Students were required to fill in weekly questions rating their knowledge and understanding about the issues covered; their satisfaction with the course; and a mood scale. This is very important aspect for us, enabling us to demonstrate impact to current and future funders. By demonstrating to students that the data was anonymised, and by explaining why we were collecting these data, we were able to gather the necessary information.
Further details	Depression Alliance Scotland, Tel: 0845 123 23 20; email: info@dascot.org; **www.dascot.org** and **www.lookokfeelcrap.org** Depression**Alliance** Scotland

LLTTF classes in schools

Practitioner	Alison Crawford and Nick Smiley, educational psychologists
Setting	Scottish Local Authority Educational Psychology Services (North Lanarkshire and East Renfrewshire)
Population	Young people aged 14–17 years in local authority secondary schools
Five Areas intervention being delivered	Living Life To The Full group work programme and training module for facilitators
How did you match what was offered to meet the person's needs?	The young people most likely to derive benefit from the programme are identified by group facilitators following training module and discussions with school pastoral support staff.
Who is supporting/ delivering this work?	Educational psychologists, home school partnership officers and school staff
How did you introduce the approach?	Educational psychologists presented the approach to colleagues and providing training for school-based staff. The approach was then presented to identified young people as a programme to build confidence and enhance wellbeing. Young people were given an option of participating in the programme.
What has gone well?	This programme is seen as very relevant to young people in secondary education. Staff working with this population believe the programme content enhances supports already available and report that it is well planned and easy to deliver. Young people report that the materials are attractive, the subject matter relevant to their everyday experiences and the strategies suggested effective in helping them develop confidence to deal with problems. They valued the experience of sharing thoughts in a group and supporting each other. Evaluations using self-report suggest that gains are made in peer group relationships, reduction in anxious feelings, social engagement and family relationships. Young people also report better concentration in class. Group work such as the LLTTF class programme provides opportunities to engage and deliver service to young women who are historically under-represented in presentation for support from educational psychology services.
What hasn't gone so well?	As this programme was originally designed for use with young adults, some of the materials were adapted to make them more suitable for the secondary school population. Activity breaks were used to pace group sessions, 'real-life' examples used to illustrate points and opportunities to revisit and refresh provided throughout the programme. It is likely that not all young people will require or may benefit from this programme. It has been our experience that careful selection of young people to be invited maximises the impact of the group.
What problems were there, and how have you worked to overcome any problems?	Some young people required individual follow-up after the group; capacity to do this should be considered during the planning stages. Usual group work issues of establishing trust and encouraging everyone to participate – these were overcome as the programme progressed.

→

What have you learned from working in this way?	The programme harnesses young people's curiosity about themselves and their peers. It provides opportunities for sharing experiences of challenging personal and social situations in a 'safe' environment and allows young people to construct positive plans for moving forward. Helping young people to understand the connections between thoughts, feelings, physical feelings and behaviour is particularly powerful.
What's been the overall impact?	• Increased confidence. • Reduction in low mood/anxious feelings. • Increased social contact. • Improved peer group and family relationships. • Greater self-awareness re: the interconnectedness of thoughts, feelings and behaviour. • Further developing school staff's understanding of issues relating to emotional wellbeing and how to support young people who are experiencing low mood and/or anxiety.
What is the single greatest benefit?	Opportunity provided to discuss issues which are very important to young people, to share experiences, to understand ourselves better and to find positive ways forward.
Any hints and tips for others?	Prepare well, take time and care selecting a group, be prepared for discussions about the 'big' issue, be flexible. The importance of the 'guided self-help' approach should be emphasised; follow up between sessions is important and facilitates the development of lasting relationships.
Further details	Alison Crawford, Depute Principal Psychologist, North Lanarkshire Council, crawfordal@northlan.gov.uk Nick Smiley, senior educational psychologist, East Renfrewshire Council, nick.smiley@eastrenfrewshire.gov.uk More information about how the programme was used is available in the PDP report 2008/2009 pp 77–137, which can be accessed at: **www.ltscotland.org.uk/pdp/index.asp**
Any other comments?	The honesty and accessibility of the programme and the quality of the resources appeals to young people.

Using the Little CBT Books in secondary schools

Name	Christabel Boyle
Setting	Secondary school in Glasgow, Scotland
Population	Pupils aged 13–14
Five Areas intervention being delivered	This was a research study to evaluate the LLTF Little CBT Books delivered as a teaching package in schools. A pilot study has been carried out to investigate the feasibility of delivering the LLTTF resources in a secondary school in Glasgow by teaching staff. Staff and pupil opinion was recorded in qualitative interviews.
How did you match what was offered to meet the person's needs?	In the pilot study each pupil (total number 280) and their teacher received one of the Little CBT Books. Teachers were also provided with lesson plans for each book and also received training of one hour, detailing the background of the study and explaining how to use the Little CBT Books.

→

Who is supporting/ delivering this work?	Teachers, education managers and educational psychology managers in Glasgow
How did you introduce the approach?	I approached the senior staff at the secondary school with the help of a liaison teacher in Child and Adolescent Mental Health Services (CAMHS) to explain the purpose of the study, show them the materials and ask for their assistance in performing the pilot. It was explained to the teachers that LLTTF books could be a very useful resource as part of their personal and social education (PSE) curriculum.
What has gone well?	The pilot study was successfully carried out in a secondary school in Glasgow and each class had one of the booklets delivered during a PSE lesson. Quantitative and qualitative feedback was obtained from pupils and teachers. Generally pupils and teachers have found the LLTTF books very interesting and useful and felt they would be a useful resource in the classroom.
What hasn't gone so well?	Some pupils did not understand the relevance of the books – and lesson plans are being revised to include relevant examples that might apply in the pupil's life now or in the future – or in the lives of those around them. The schools was reluctant to pilot mental health questionnaires, which means an alternative school has had to be found for this part of the study.
What problems were there, and how have you worked to overcome any problems?	Problem as mentioned above, i.e. piloting mental health questionnaires, but another school has been found for this. Discussion about how LLTTF resource might help schools achieve the health and wellbeing outcomes of 'Curriculum for Excellence' encourages schools to take part in the study. There was the problem of anonymity: the secondary school felt unable to give pupils an ID number and give out generic questionnaires for evaluation accordingly. (The pupils had to complete two questionnaires, one before and after the lesson.) Therefore the research team had to ask pupils to put their names on the questionnaires which were then removed and put into a password-protected Excel database and exchanged for ID numbers.
What have you learned from working in this way?	Books for the teaching can be delivered as a lesson by the teacher in the classroom of a secondary school and they are acceptable to the teachers and pupils.
What's been the overall impact?	There has been enthusiasm from the teachers for this new resource and due to a successful pilot the work can progress on to the next phase which will ultimately conclude with a randomised controlled trial evaluating LLTTF in the classroom.
What is the single greatest benefit?	Hopefully the greatest benefit will be improved mood amongst secondary school pupils in Glasgow but this is still to be evaluated.
Any hints and tips for others?	In order to raise the interest of teachers and encourage their willingness to participate in LLTTF it might be useful to discuss how the course might help the school achieve the health and wellbeing outcomes of 'Curriculum for Excellence'.
Further details	christabel.boyle@nhs.net

Living Life to the Full free online course (www.llttf.com)

Practitioner	Liz Rafferty, WISH Programme manager
Setting	The WISH Programme works with three health board areas across Scotland and with Depression Alliance Scotland in a pilot supporting the Living Life to the Full Interactive package.
Population	Mild to moderate depression and anxiety in settings mainly outwith the NHS.
Five Areas intervention being delivered	Small training teams have been appointed in each health board area. All of the leads and trainers have been trained in the Five Areas approach by the programme manager. The trainers then go on to train interested organisations in their locality. The main goal is to widen access to an effective evidence-based intervention. In addition Depression Alliance Scotland is supporting the use of the Living Life to the Full Interactive package. Again, the aim is to allow open access to this website with support across Scotland.
How did you match what was offered to meet the person's needs?	Each area will be able to provide a range of materials such as classes, large book, small book, DVDs and websites. The trainers will discuss with the interested parties which resources will best meet their needs and provide the relevant training in how best to use them with their clients. In the case of the Living Life to the Full Interactive package individuals contact Depression Alliance Scotland themselves after seeing an advert in local press or linked websites.
Who is supporting/ delivering this work?	There have been a range of organisations who have already taken up the option of being trained in the Five Areas approach such as Back-to-Work agencies, Social Work, Women's Aid, Building Healthy Communities, Lesbian, Gay, Bisexual and Transgender, GPs, OTs, Older Adult Services. In the Depression Alliance Scotland pilot there is a support worker to help people get the most out of the Living Life to the Full Interactive package.
How did you introduce the approach?	The trainers meet with the local interested teams and give an overview of the approach and how this can be used with their clients. In the case of the Depression Alliance Scotland pilot once someone makes contact they are given information about what the package and support will involve to help them decide if they want to participate.
What has gone well?	The programme is only in the early stages with training of teams commencing in January 2010. Even so there has been no shortage of interested teams and each area now has a training programme in place. Feedback from those who have received the training thus far has been positive, with trainees finding the training very valuable and applicable to their clients. User feedback has also been positive. So far there have been steady numbers of interested people for the Depression Alliance Scotland pilot.

→

What hasn't gone so well?	It has taken longer than anticipated to get the programme running for a variety of reasons. Staff recruitment took longer than anticipated, Training of the trainers was delayed and also adverse weather conditions have impacted on delivery of the training.
What problems were there – and how have you worked to overcome any problems?	A particular issue was ensuring that training packages would be suitable for the trainees. Some areas felt that their needs were different for their population. Therefore there was significant work undertaken with the local teams, in conjunction with Professor Chris Williams to have a variety of training materials available. In terms of the Depression Alliance Scotland pilot the initial plan was not to have people with a score of >21 on the PHQ 9 taking part but there has been a number of people who have been scoring >21 showing an interest. We have therefore put into place a protocol to ensure that people are not actively suicidal, are seeing their GP, the GP has agreed to them taking part and that they have a suitable safety plan in place.
What have you learned from working in this way?	From the training perspective it has become clear that the approach has wide application across a range of services and age ranges and that there has been a great interest from agencies out with the NHS to deliver an effective evidenced based intervention. With regard to the Depression Alliance Scotland pilot there is already evidence that people are interested in working online as a way of improving how they feel.
What's been the overall impact?	As yet the training programme has not had enough time to establish an impact level. The impact is expected to increase significantly as the programme develops. There are early signs within the Depression Alliance Scotland pilot of significant improvement in both PHQ 9 and GAD 7 scores.
What is the single greatest benefit?	I think the single greatest benefit in both the training and the Depression Alliance Scotland pilot is the way that the Five Areas has been received by the trainees and individuals using the package. The approach seems to fit very well with the experiences people have had and they are able to apply the approach in their everyday life.
Any hints and tips for others?	The key component to people benefiting from the approach is the support that is offered. The most important thing is to be very knowledgeable about the materials when using them and to have enthusiasm.
Further details	Liz Rafferty; Tel: 0141 232 0013; email: liz.rafferty@ggc.scot.nhs.uk

Living Life to the Full Interactive (www.llttfi.com) offered across Scotland (pilot service)

Practitioner	Susanne Dick, low intensity practitioner, Edinburgh, UK
Setting	Scotland-wide intervention delivered by Depression Alliance Scotland
Population	We are looking to support 500 people over age 18 throughout the course duration (September 2009 to end March 2011). We are delivering the service Scotland-wide and are particularly targeting people who are less likely to reach out for help and support through traditional services.
Five Areas intervention being delivered	Living Life to the Full Interactive (LLTTFi) is a computerised CBT course delivered individually over six to eight weeks with one-to-one telephone support. The course has six structured sessions covering common problems such as unhelpful thinking, reduced activity, sleeping problems, low confidence, etc. Each session has an accompanying workbook, which is available to download from the website. This is being delivered as part of a national public health initiative called WISH funded by the Scottish government. The overall aim is to widen access to an effective evidence-based intervention for people who experience mild to moderate depression and or anxiety. Increasing access to psychological therapies can also provide an alternative to antidepressant prescribing.
How did you match what was offered to meet the person's needs?	A primary purpose of this course is to enable people to work on issues and problems they face in their own lives. This is done in two ways. In the first session, participants are asked to fill in a questionnaire about their mood and areas of difficulty. The online course then puts this information together to prioritise the modules they complete during the six weeks. This means that they work on the issues that are most relevant to them. Secondly, the sessions and worksheets are written in a way so that participants will practise techniques on their own examples rather than generic examples.
Who is delivering this work?	The intervention is delivered by the Depression Alliance Scotland self-help support worker.
How did you introduce the approach?	LLTTFi is a new service for DAS and we are advertising widely in Scotland through various media and organisations. As with other services we focus on community-based advertising to attract people who might not otherwise be receiving any support or treatment for their depression. We have linked from **www.dascot.org** and **www.lookokfeelcrap.org** and have placed ads in national media such as: *The Scotsman, Inverness Courier*, the *Big Issue*, as well as establishing contact with colleges and universities and GP's. This will be a ongoing process to continually attract new participants.
What has gone well?	The planning of materials and progression through the course prior to participants starting onto the course. Most initial participants have found the interactive programme engaging and indications so far are that the majority are completing their course.
What hasn't gone so well?	It has taken more time than anticipated to do advertising and email/mail shots to generate a steady flow of participants to the service. Also, some people have taken longer than 6-8 weeks to complete the course, and have requested more time between some sessions to allow them to reflect on what they have learned before moving on. It's not a problem, just something to bear in mind!

→

What problems were there, and how have you worked to overcome any problems?	Being an online course there were initial technical problems, with occasional minor problems continuing to arise for some people. These were resolved after discussing problems with Media Innovations who were helpful and quick to resolve them. This could be a potential reason for people to drop out or present another barrier for them and it is important to resolve these issues quickly for the participant.
What have you learned from working in this way?	The importance of the telephone support in keeping people motivated. People could easily give up with online self-help material if not supported, particularly in the initial stages of course. The support can be short: we give around 100 minutes of support over the duration of the course. Also, how effective the Five Areas model can actually be and the difference it can make to people in understanding about depression/anxiety and particularly in relation to their situation and experiences.
What's been the overall impact?	Those who have already completed the course have indicated that the course has helped them understand about low mood and anxiety. It has helped them to tackle problems, particularly unhelpful thoughts. The nature of the interactive course means that we have people ranging from age 20–70 participating, located throughout Scotland. The Five Areas diagram was very powerful; people expressed shock and surprise at seeing *their* situation in front of them. People found it very useful to see how the key areas of their life are linked; this leads to understanding and helped people to begin challenging negative thoughts. Most people have said the points on the do/don'ts card have offered an effective way of helping them do this.
What is the single greatest benefit?	To be able to offer a service that can make a significant difference to people's lives whatever their geographical location within Scotland. That the service includes direct support via telephone sessions enhances this significantly. Participants to date cover the Central Belt, Fife, Dumfries, Borders, Inverness, Skye and Lewis.
Any hints and tips for others?	Be very familiar with the material: both online and the accompanying resources. Also, most people seem to reach a point where they want more time before moving on, to go back over materials, to reflect. It has been important to allow this to ensure each participant continues and has a positive, beneficial experience. It is important that delivering the course offers some flexibility to accommodate this.
Further details	Depression Alliance Scotland, Tel: 0845 123 23 20; email: info@dascot.org; **www.dascot.org** and **www.lookokfeelcrap.org** Check out the LLTTFi demo at **www.dasllttfi.co.uk** DepressionAlliance Scotland

Overcoming Bulimia Online (www.overcomingbulimiaonline.com) delivered in a specialist eating disorders service

Practitioner	Miriam Grover
Setting	London-based community outpatient psychotherapy service
Population	Specialist eating disorder research and treatment service across South-East London. Treating patients with eating disorders between the ages of 17 and 65. Approximately 450 new referrals per year.
Five Areas intervention being delivered	Overcoming Bulimia (OB) package: CD-Rom and online package being delivered to patients with bulimia/bulimic symptoms.
How did you match what was offered to meet the person's needs?	All patients are given an initial assessment of their symptoms and the assessor would discuss treatment options (including OB) with those patients with bulimia/ bulimic symptoms.
Who is supporting/ delivering this work?	OB has been supported by all clinicians in the department. Providing support for patients using the intervention has also been a useful training aid for trainee and junior staff who are early in their psychotherapy training. Support has been offered in face to face sessions, on the telephone and via email.
How did you introduce the approach?	Following initial assessment of the patient's mental and physical health, OB was introduced to all patients with bulimic symptoms who were not in need of emergency treatment due to their physical and/or mental state. Patients were given a description of the intervention and information on the evidence base regarding the efficacy of the intervention. Those patients who expressed an interest were offered the option of seeing the introduction to the package in the department. Written information to take away was also available. Patients were informed that they were able to use the package whilst waiting to start psychotherapy and were also able to use it during therapy if they wished. Patients were made aware that using the intervention would not delay the start of their psychotherapy and that if they refused the intervention then this would not have a negative impact on their access to psychotherapy. We found that this 'soft sell' of the intervention helped to reduce potential resistance to the intervention as some patients can feel 'fobbed off' by the offer of a self-help treatment.
What has gone well?	There has been high uptake of the intervention – the reasons for this being the 'user-friendly' nature of the intervention and also the ability to access treatment immediately. This level of acceptability increased further when the service changed from the CD-Rom version to the online version (OBO) of the intervention. The unlimited access of an internet-based version meant that the intervention could be accessed by patients at any time of day (or night!) and that access could be gained at home/other acceptable venue. This means that treatment was not restricted to those people who are able to take time away from work/study/family commitments in order to attend clinic appointments.
What hasn't gone so well?	Staff members needed time to understand the programme and how it could be used before they would recommend it to patients. Some patients felt 'fobbed off' by the suggestion of starting treatment with self-help.

→

What problems were there, and how have you worked to overcome any problems?	When initially establishing the intervention within the clinical setting it was important to establish a set of protocols and guidelines for the safe use of the intervention. The guidelines covered areas such as: who would provide the support; how often support would be provided; how clinical risk would be managed; and what action would be taken in the event of loss of contact with the patient or in the event of a crisis. The aims of providing these guidelines were to ensure that staff members were aware of what was required of them and their responsibilities to the patients were clear and that patients were aware of the service they were receiving whilst using the intervention and where to turn if they were experiencing difficulties. Initially we were using the CD-Rom version of OB; patients would attend the clinic in order to use the intervention and would be met by clinic staff as they attended 'appointments' to use the intervention and clinicians were 'on hand' should the patient express any difficulties. When using the CD-Rom version, it was important to ensure that patients did not enter any identifying information on the programme due to data protection issues should the computer be stolen. Our clinic decided to use the online version of the intervention (OBO) when this became available because our patient population often had work, study or childcare commitments. Often patients said they were able to secure time for appointments for therapy but that they would not be able to take time out to complete a self-help treatment as well as time out for therapy, even though they wanted to use OB. One of the major difficulties in providing an online treatment intervention within a clinical setting is minimising risk with patients whom clinicians may not be seeing on a regular basis, i.e. those patients using OBO whilst waiting to start face to face therapy. When the service changed from using the CD-Rom version of the intervention to OBO, these guidelines had to be reviewed to account for the fact that patients would now be using the intervention at home rather than in the clinic.
What have you learned from working in this way?	It is possible to use self-help treatments as one of a repertoire of treatments in a specialist clinic. Patients find computerised self-help treatments to be acceptable and effective in helping them.
What's been the overall impact?	Many patients have used the OB package and patient satisfaction has been high. Some patients have not required any further treatment after having used OB and many patients have reported lowered symptom levels after having used the package. Patients felt that OB had helped them to understand the illness and how to combat it.
What is the single greatest benefit?	Being able to offer patients treatment immediately and in a flexible way that suits them.
Any hints and tips for others?	Take time as a team to discuss how using an intervention such as this would work within your own clinical setting. To ensure that the intervention is recommended appropriately, it is important that all staff are familiar with the programme and its contents. It is very important that staff are given the time and space to express and discuss any concerns about 'being replaced by a computer'. Ensure that you have a set of guidelines for your staff so that everyone is aware of what their responsibilities are and so that risk is managed adequately.
Further details	miriam.grover@kcl.ac.uk

Overcoming Anorexia Online (www.overcominganorexiaonline.com) delivered in a specialist eating disorders clinic

Practitioners	Lubna Mohammad-Dar, Dannie Glennon and Miriam Grover, psychologist and psychotherapists
Setting	London-based community outpatient psychotherapy service
Population	Specialist eating disorder research and treatment service across South-East London. Treating patients with eating disorders between the ages of 17 and 65. Approximately 450 new referrals per year.
Five Areas intervention being delivered	Overcoming Anorexia Online (OAO; a CBT-based intervention for carers of people with anorexia that is accessed via the internet) was used within the department as part of a clinical research programme investigating effective treatments for people with anorexia nervosa and their carers. Carers of people referred to the department for assessment and treatment of anorexia were invited to take part in the study, either directly (if they attended the patient's assessment appointment) or they were contacted indirectly by letter, phone or email (with the patient's permission) if they did not attend the assessment appointment. For the purpose of the study, consenting carers were randomised to either OAO or a control support intervention (provided by beat: **www.b-eat.co.uk**).
How did you match what was offered to meet the person's needs?	Carers were asked if they felt they needed to gain greater understanding of anorexia and how it affects their loved one, help to develop practical skills in their caring role and whether they felt they needed practical and emotional support in their caring role. Those carers who felt that this might be of benefit to them were invited to join the study. We did however check with the carers that they were not suffering from significant mental health problems themselves (such as depression, psychosis or substance misuse) that might mean that they should prioritise their own needs before embarking on assisting their loved one to combat anorexia.
Who is supporting/ delivering this work?	The research project was led by MG. LM-D and DG provided the clinical support for all carers randomised to OAO. This consisted of weekly contact via phone or email while they were completing the intervention and monthly contact during the follow-up period.
How did you introduce the approach?	All carers were sent a welcome letter on the study including information leaflets, contact information and further details on the intervention they were randomised to. Carers randomised to the control support intervention by beat were given information on how to access beat's services and were asked to keep a diary of how often they contacted beat and the purpose of each contact. Carers assigned to OAO were sent detailed information about how to access the intervention including a log-in name and password. Following this, those carers randomised to OAO were emailed an introduction to their support therapist and were offered the option of having either telephone or email support depending on their needs and preferences.
What has gone well?	Carers randomised to OAO reported that they liked the OAO intervention as it gave them practical tools that they could use in their everyday caring role. They also liked to use the workbooks to revisit the most salient points of each module. Carers using the OAO intervention also gave feedback that they valued the support given, either by phone or email. Quoting (with permission) from a carer who was randomised to OAO: 'As well as the programme contents, which are really useful, just having someone to encourage and praise me has been a huge support.' Carers who received the control support intervention generally gave feedback that it was useful to have somebody at the end of a phone, and to be able to access information off the website including the message board online.

→

What hasn't gone so well?	Carers commented that sometimes they found it difficult to allow themselves protected time to log on to OAO. However, they found it useful to print out the workbooks, giving them more flexibility in being able to access the material. Carers who received support from beat said that they would have liked access to a 24-hour telephone support line. They also commented that there is a lack of support groups in some areas of the country.
What problems were there, and how have you worked to overcome any problems?	All carers using OAO had difficulties initially logging on to the program. All new logins will be generated for future use to remedy this difficulty. Services using OAO need to acknowledge that support therapists need dedicated time during their working day in which to give support. We would suggest that a dedicated one-hour slot would enable a therapist to support three carers.
What have you learned from working in this way?	It is vital that carers feel supported whilst a loved one is in treatment. As a service trying to meet the needs of all our carers in line with NICE guidelines, due to the success of the initial trial of OAO in our department, we are now planning to offer OAO to all carers of people with anorexia as part of the treatment package.
What's been the overall impact?	In our experience carers felt empowered with skills and confidence to support the sufferer. The OAO intervention proved a useful tool in being able to impart knowledge, skills and support on a national and international basis, where often support for carers is very limited.
What is the single greatest benefit?	As a service it provides flexibility in working with carers in a different medium. For carers it enables them to grow in confidence in being able to support their loved ones.
Any hints and tips for others?	Different carers may have different needs in terms of support but these will probably fall into the following categories: • Need for encouragement to continue caring. • Need to establish boundaries around the sufferer's behaviour. • Need to establish boundaries around the carer's caring behaviour. • Advice on how to deal with a particular situation or behaviour. • Need to 'off-load'. Remember that email communication does not have any contextual cues that one gets with verbal communication, so it is important that you ensure that your message is clear and is unlikely to be misinterpreted. The support given is not formal counselling but should encompass fundamental 'counselling skills', e.g. a non-judgmental approach, warmth, genuineness. Activities such as information giving and 'expert advice' are part of the role of the supporter and can be given if these are sought by the carer.
Further details	South London and Maudsley NHS NHS Foundation Trust Lubna Mohammad-Dar: lubna.mohammad@slam.nhs.uk Dannie Glennon: dannie.glennon@slam.nhs.uk Tel: 0203 228 3180 Miriam Grover: miriam.grover@kcl.ac.uk

Self-help clinic in a primary care mental health team

Name	Michelle McAuley, Glasgow, Scotland
Setting	Primary care mental health team
Population	Adults
Five Areas intervention being delivered	Patients were given the choice of using either the *Overcoming depression and low mood* workbooks posted to them (Williams 2006) or the free online www.livinglifetothefull.com website.
How did you match what was offered to meet the person's needs?	The CBT-Self-Help (CBT-SH) pathway began at the weekly referral meeting where appropriate patients were selected by the team. Patients were sent an information letter about the CBT-SH service, a PHQ-9 and a PHQ-7 and an opt-in sheet. Persons who opted into the CBT-SH service completed a brief (approximately eight minutes) telephone assessment to ensure suitability for the CBT-SH. Suitable persons were informed of who their support worker was and when their first support session would occur and that they would either have their workbooks posted to them or the web address emailed to them.
Who is supporting/ delivering this work?	With regards to who delivered the support, this involved two team members with very different backgrounds. One was a trained professional (CBT therapist) and the other was a para-professional trained in offering supported self-help. They had both achieved a level of competency to offer support and had attended the SPIRIT CBT self-help training course [see Chapter 11].
How did you introduce the approach?	Introducing a new element of service in an existing team can be a challenge, and aligning the new service with the team objectives is important. Prior to the intervention, we conducted meetings with the team. In devising the intervention, there were considerations regarding the administrative side of introducing the intervention that also needed to take into account the existing structures, such as screening procedures, establishing risk protocols, and issues of support and supervision. Overall, involving the existing team in the implementation of the new service, gives a sense of ownership to the team, and generates greater involvement and support for the intervention.
What has gone well?	The current model has proved to be a feasible intervention within a primary mental health care team, and fully adaptable within the stepped care model. One of the strengths of the intervention has been the opportunity to offer patients a choice of interventions, which were of immediate access.
What hasn't gone so well?	A challenge is how to bring about sustained use of the approach. Some practitioners avoid the training or bring negative views about the idea/ concept of using self-help and low intensity ways of working.

→

What problems were there, and how have you worked to overcome any problems?	Throughout the development of the guided CBT service there were a number of challenges the team faced. • Risk assessment: The use of question 9 from the PHQ-9 proved to be challenging as although it clearly identifies thoughts regarding suicide there is little scope to ascertain if the patient is planning to act on these thoughts. Thus to ensure that persons at risk to themselves were only excluded we used two risk questions initially and once support had been established. • Staff arrangements: Important in all service redesign; staff are an integral force for the success of the project. Therefore there was a need to provide training and support for staff offering support including the wider team as well as the two initial workers delivering the intervention. Supervision was provided for support workers and training in the materials and how to offer support. Staff concerns were primarily regarding issues of risk and when/if the service would be inappropriate for patients. Risk was addressed by providing a clear and concise risk protocol and supervision. Pre-selection of new referrals was initially offered to allow staff members to remain confident in the project. However, as confidence grew within one month the team agreed that all new referrals would be invited to opt into the supported CBT-SH service.
What have you learned from working in this way?	The resources needed to run this project, once it is set up, are quite minimal. We have estimated a total of 75 minutes per client including both therapy and administration time; the intervention has great potential to help reducing overall therapy time, waiting lists and patient satisfaction.
What's been the overall impact?	An audit of the outcomes of the referrals period between 1 November 2007 and 12 February 2008 included 99 invites, and 37 persons opted in. Of the 37 who opted in, 32 engaged with the supported self-help service (86.5 per cent). Of those who engaged with the service 68 per cent were female. The mean age was 42 years old. With regards to the mental health of the pilot sample, the mean PHQ-9 score was 13.9 and the mean PHQ-7 score was 12.3; 55 per cent of the sample were not currently using prescribed medication for their mental illness; and only 38.7 per cent had used self-help before in treating their difficulties. We received 16/30 (53 per cent) of the follow-up data at approximately six weeks. 62.5 per cent (10) completed the six support sessions. The mean scores before the guided self-help service or the PHQ-9 and GAD-7 was 14.1 and 12.4, respectively, and after the guided self-help service the mean scores were 7.8 and 6.5. A paired t-test was performed and the mean difference in the PHQ-9 depression scores was 6.33 (p-value < 0.005; 95 per cent confidence interval –3.623 to 9.044). The paired t-test for the GAD7 anxiety score provided a mean difference of 5.933 (p-value <0.005; 95 per cent confidence interval 3.307 to 8.560). For both scores the difference was positive showing a marked improvement in both depression and anxiety levels for clients. Of the 16 providing follow up data, 11 (68.8 per cent) had not received any other support for their mental health difficulties or had accessed any other self-help material.
What is the single greatest benefit?	Marked improvement in both depression and anxiety levels for clients.
Any hints and tips for others?	• Provide patients with choice of materials. • Offering a blanket opt-in to all new referrals rather than pre-selection of patients.
Further details	Michelle McAuley: mmcauley@nhs.net

PART 6

Supporter scripts and resources

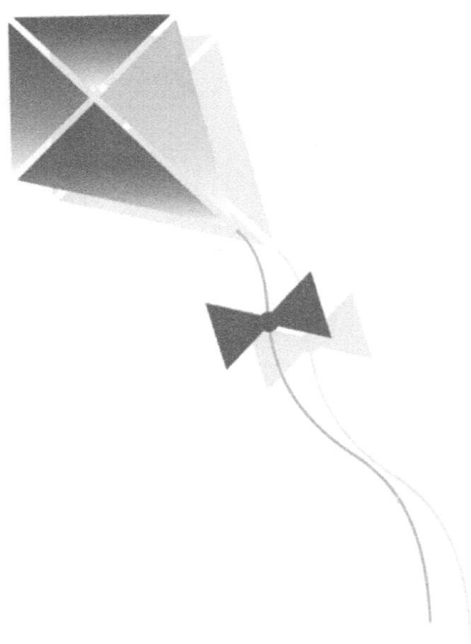

Dr Chris Williams

www.livinglifetothefull.com/www.llttf.com
www.llttfi.com
www.fiveareas.com

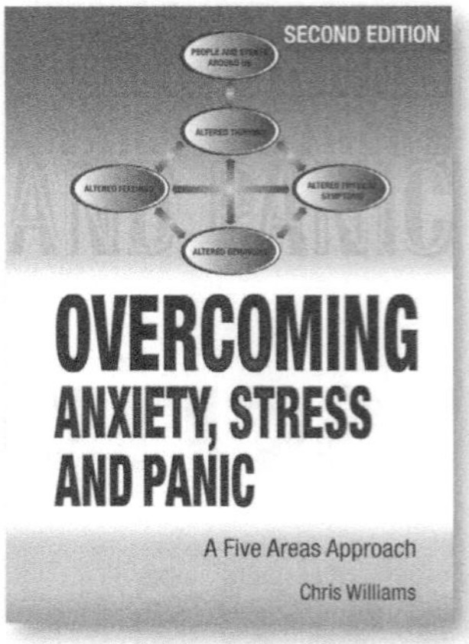
SECOND EDITION
OVERCOMING
ANXIETY, STRESS
AND PANIC
A Five Areas Approach
Chris Williams

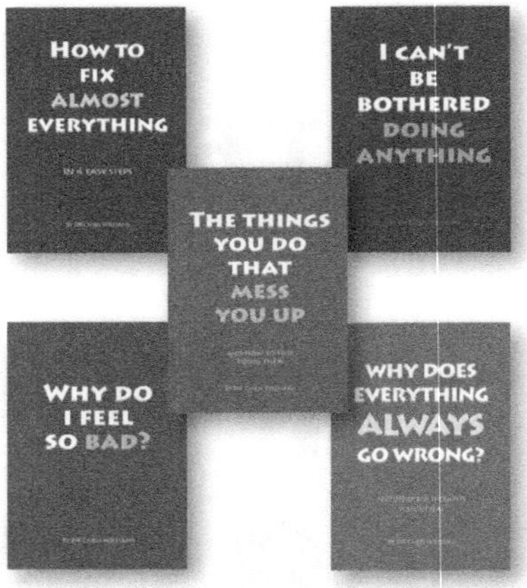
HOW TO FIX ALMOST EVERYTHING
I CAN'T BE BOTHERED DOING ANYTHING
THE THINGS YOU DO THAT MESS YOU UP
WHY DO I FEEL SO BAD?
WHY DOES EVERYTHING ALWAYS GO WRONG?

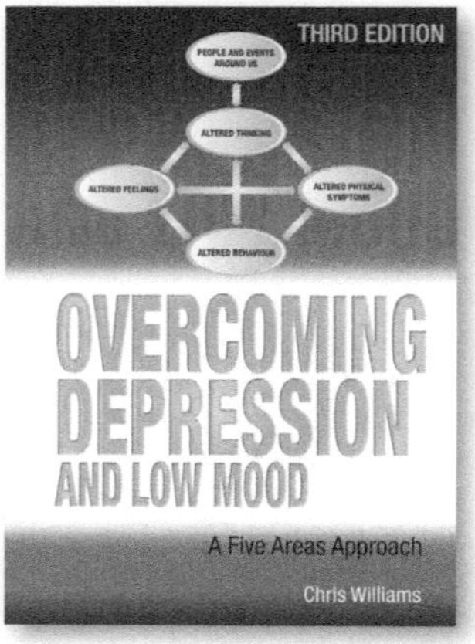
THIRD EDITION
OVERCOMING
DEPRESSION
AND LOW MOOD
A Five Areas Approach
Chris Williams

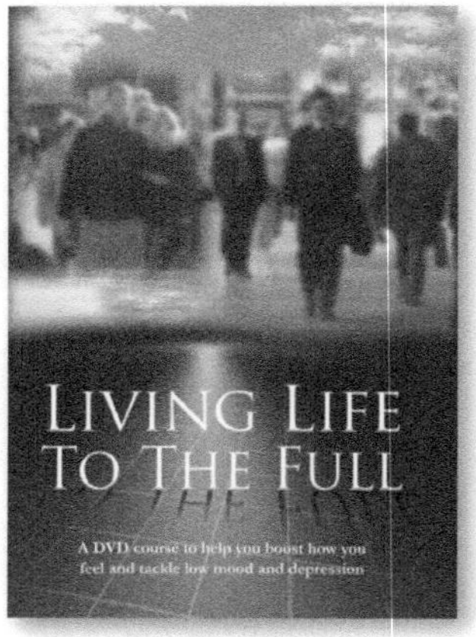
LIVING LIFE
TO THE FULL
A DVD course to help you boost how you feel and tackle low mood and depression

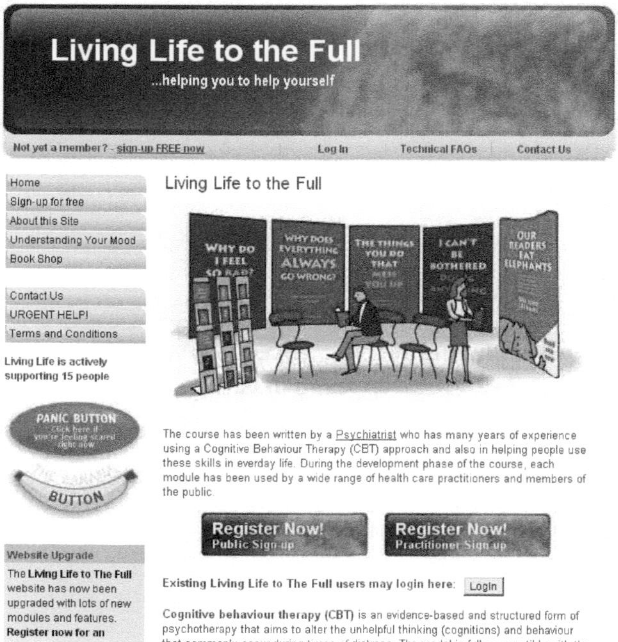
Living Life to the Full
...helping you to help yourself
Not yet a member? - sign-up FREE now
Log In
Technical FAQs
Contact Us
Home
Sign-up for free
About this Site
Understanding Your Mood
Book Shop
Contact Us
URGENT HELP!
Terms and Conditions
Living Life is actively supporting 15 people
PANIC BUTTON
BUTTON
Website Upgrade
The Living Life to The Full website has now been upgraded with lots of new modules and features. Register now for an
Living Life to the Full
The course has been written by a Psychiatrist who has many years of experience using a Cognitive Behaviour Therapy (CBT) approach and also in helping people use these skills in everday life. During the development phase of the course, each module has been used by a wide range of health care practitioners and members of the public.
Register Now! Public Sign-up
Register Now! Practitioner Sign-up
Existing Living Life to The Full users may login here:
Login
Cognitive behaviour therapy (CBT) is an evidence-based and structured form of psychotherapy that aims to alter the unhelpful thinking (cognitions) and behaviour

1 Contents

1 Contents 219
2 Introduction to using these resources 220
3 Planner sheet 221
4 Review sheet 222
5 Supporters, key points checklist face to face support 224
6 Telephone supporters, key points checklist 228
7 Further information and resources 233

2 Introduction to using these resources

These resources are designed to help you introduce, support and review your patients'/clients' work using the various **Five Areas** resources.

The Five Areas Assessment model is designed to help people better understand how their thoughts, feelings, physical symptoms, behaviour and environmental factors can unhelpfully affect their mental health. Once the initial Five Areas assessment workbook (*Understanding why I feel...*) has been completed, you can work together to identify ways to alter any problems identified.

To help the person make changes, a range of smaller and larger written resources, DVD and online websites are available. Together, these provide a comprehensive modular self-help programme based on a structured form of psychotherapy (CBT). This approach has been devised to help people who are experiencing mild to moderate depression and anxiety.

Working in this way can encourage people to take greater responsibility for discoveries about their problems, and lead to a sense of empowerment.

Suggested support:

- Send out or give a **Welcome pack** (Envelope 1) of key support resources. This includes the **Starting out ...** workbook – i.e. how to work using the approach.
- Arrange a next appointment time and encourage the client to read the **Starting out ...** workbook in advance if they can.
- At your first full support session, go through how you will work together on their problems and ask the person to plan to complete the **Understanding why you feel as you do** workbook (i.e. the Five Areas assessment) by the next session.
- A checklist in this handout outlines the topics to cover in introducing and then reviewing progress.
- Use the two key **Planner** and **Review** sheets in this handout to help the person. **Plan, Do and Review.**
- The person can then choose to work on any other workbooks/modules in any order – however, we suggest the reduced activity, sleep, and medication management modules are especially appropriate first choices.
- Envelope 2 contains additional planner/review resources and can be sent out or given together with the next one to two key intervention workbooks.
- Regular short review contacts allow you to encourage, review and support the person in working in this way.

3 Planner sheet

My Notes **Date**

Which workbook/module will I work on next?

Plan to take things forwards

1). **What** am I going to do?

2). **When** am I going to do it?

Is my planned task one that:

Q) Will be useful for understanding or changing how I am?	Yes	No
Q) Is a specific task so that I will know when I have done it?	Yes	No
Q) Is realistic: is it practical and achievable?	Yes	No

3). What problems/difficulties could arise, and how can I overcome this?

Mood rating score: (date)

My next contact time ....

Re-arrangement details: Remember – if you know in advance you can't make the session, please let us know by contacting your local support worker

PLEASE NOTE: If you are struggling/feel worse, or if at any time you feel suicidal please visit your doctor/go to A+E/phone NHS 24/ NHS Direct

4 Review sheet

For discussion dated:

What task (s) had you planned to do?

Write it here

Did you attempt the task? Yes No

If yes:

- What went well?
- What didn't go so well?
- What have you learned about from what happened?
- How are you going to apply what you have learned?

If not:

What stopped you?

- My internal factors (e.g. forgot, not enough time, put it off, concerns I couldn't do it, I couldn't see the point of it, etc.).
- External factors (events that happened, work/home issues, etc.).
- How could you have planned to tackle these blocks?

5 Supporters' key points for checklist for face to face support

At every session: Building an effective working relationship

1	**Communications**
	Collaborative agenda: relevant to them
	The presence of a focus and clear structure to the session – cut through confusion – clear things to do
	Focus on the materials – and motivating/planning change
2	**Collaborative relationship**
	Practitioner encouraging the patient to participate fully through questioning techniques, shared problem-solving and decision making, etc.
	Adequate time for the patient to answer questions
	Repeatedly link back progress and targets being worked on to the Five Areas assessment
	Restate: making changes in any area will lead to benefits in other areas in life
3	**Communication skills**
	Put at ease. Show warmth, empathy and genuineness
	Checking/clarified and summarised what was said
	Pacing – so that the session doesn't seem rushed
4	**Plan, Do, Review model**
	Jointly agreed
	Clear, specific plan

First contact

1	**Brief introductory contact**	**Tick**
	Welcome pack given or sent to people before first support appointment **Contents**: Your service details sheet (as available) Support worker details (as available) Copy of ***Starting out*** workbook or ***Why do I feel so bad*** book Mood Scale (as used in your service – though we recommend a mood scale combining the PHQ9 and GAD7)	
	Complete a brief learning evaluation: *We have various support options available. We'll talk more about these next time. Can I ask though – are you the sort of person who:* – *Likes more detail and really understand things?* – *Prefers just key to-the-point instructions?* – *Likes TV documentaries with real-life people talking about how they cope with things?* – *Do you have access to a DVD/broadband computer?*	
	Based on what you've told me, I'd recommend x, y Provide appropriate start-up materials for that recommendation, i.e. Ask to read *Starting out/ Write all over your bathroom mirror* and/or one of the LLTTF DVD (suggest watch introduction module) or LLTTF starter sheet – and to complete mood scales in advance of first appointment if they can	

Main support sessions

2	**First main session of support**	
2a	Introduction – you/them – check names to use	
	Do you have a pen and paper?	
	Explain there may be some pauses as you make notes	
	Complete initial assessment as you usually would	
	Brief mention of the Five Areas approach – to help summarise key problems – and help decide together what you will work on changing	
	Briefly point out that ***Understanding why you feel/ Why do I feel so bad*** book you will give today will help them find out more about how low mood is affecting them – and how to change things for the better	
	Repeat **Mood Scale** now and link to reviewing progress/compare with their ratings	
2b	**Introduction to the CBT approach**	
	Link this workbook approach with the person's own specific mentioned problems (workbooks and modules will help you tackle the … xxx)	
	Cognitive behavioural therapy – what it means – avoid jargon	
	What you will learn (practical life skills addressing your problems) – a treatment of choice (NICE/national treatment guidelines)	

→

2c	**Clarify choice of resource**	
	Complete a learning evaluation (if not completed at first contact): *Are you the sort of person who:* – *Likes more detail and really understand things?* – *Prefers just key to-the-point instructions?* – *Likes TV documentaries with real-life people talking about how they cope with things?* – *Do you have access to a DVD/broadband computer?* *Based on what you've told me, I'd recommend x, y for you* **If have access to a computer** now talk through a quick overview of the LLTTF site and key features. Sign them up for the reminder newsletters. Show the forum and consider a trial post (hello I'm new). Option of a support association	
	Based on what you told me before, I recommend that XX resource will suit how you want to work Briefly flick through key elements of the first resource ***Understanding why you feel/Why do I feel so bad*** (5 mins)	
2d	**Working together with a plan**	
	Describe total number of support sessions/time available (e.g. 4–6 contacts of up to 2 hours in total – or whatever time is available – e.g. 20 minute supports within our usual sessions)	
	Common and normal to feel de-motivated – or to find change difficult to start with	
	Therefore we will work together – regular support/motivate	
2e	**Goals**	
	We'll check progress each session using a Mood checklist – show and option to complete	
	Aim is to help you '*turn the corner*'.	
	If by the end of the support you still feel you need extra support/treatments we can discuss that with your GP/other workers	
2f	**Next steps using the resources – other session(s)**	
	First step is to find out more about why you feel as you do/get started	
	Point to the *Understanding why you feel as you do* workbook to be used first	
	Identify key points that workbook will cover (i.e. Why do I feel so bad?) – Plus first online module in **www.llttf.com** (*Starting out)* if they wish/*DVD Introduction*	
	Make a clear plan for what to do next – using the **Planner sheet** (introduce) and focus on planning to use the *Understanding why I feel …* workbook	
2g	**Ending the session**	
	Quick summary recap of key points	
	Confirm a time and number for the next call/contact	
	Reminder there is a practice task at the end – important to carry out	
	Encourage/praise/motivate and brief review of what actions agreed to do this week	
	End	

Follow-up sessions checklist: reviewing and planning

1	**Welcome back and scene setting**	
	Text reminder a day before appointment/on the day (optional)	
	Nice to see/hear you again – we have about x (usually 20) minutes again this session	
	Brief overview of this session (we'll check how your using the approach is going, discuss your mood scores, choose a next target to focus on and then make a plan of how to do that). Is that okay?	
	Doesn't matter if there have been problems/didn't like it – I'm here just to check and help	
	Have you been able to complete the **Review sheet**?	
	Have you been able to complete the **Mood rating**? Go through outcome and record. Respond with team risk response if positive risk item.	
2	**Use of the approach this week**	
	Review experience of using/not the materials using the structure on the **Review sheet**	
	Have you used them – if yes – praise If no – look at blocks from **Review sheet** – and problem solve solutions (problems are common – great opportunity to learn)	
	Choose to stick/apply current workbook – or choose to cover new resources/worksheets or modules as needed – and give brief overview/rationale • Good initial topics to focus on are reduced activity/can't be bothered doing anything • Sleep/medication concordance	
	Agree a clear plan for what to do using **Planner sheet**	
3	**Ending the session**	
	Quick summary recap of key points	
	Confirm a time and number for the next call/contact 30 minute window	
	Encourage/praise/motivate and brief review of what actions agreed to do this week	

6 Telephone supporters' key points checklist

At every session: Building an effective working relationship

1	**Communications**
	Collaborative agenda: relevant to them
	The presence of a focus and clear structure to the session – cut through confusion – clear things to do
	Focus on the materials – and motivating/planning change
2	**Collaborative relationship**
	Practitioner encouraging the patient to participate fully through questioning techniques, shared problem-solving and decision making, etc.
	Adequate time for the patient to answer questions
	Repeatedly link back progress and targets being worked on to the Five Areas assessment
	Restate: making changes in any area will lead to benefits in other areas in life
3	**Communication skills**
	Put at ease: show warmth, empathy and genuineness
	Checking/clarified and summarised what was said
	Pacing – so that the session doesn't seem rushed
4	**Plan, Do, Review model**
	Jointly agreed
	Clear, specific plan

Introductory session checklist

		Tick
0	**Welcome pack sent to people before first support appointment** **Contents**: Your Support Worker Details/Welcome to the service Mood Scale Copy of Big Books (***Starting out*** and ***Understanding why I feel as I do***) workbooks or Little Books ***Why do I feel so Bad*** and ***Write all over your Bathroom Mirror*** or details of website used **Request to read Starting out/Write all over …**	
1	**Initial short appointment arranging telephone contact**	
	Patient phones to book appointment – or otherwise you initiate contact	
	Brief Introductions – you/them – agree names to use	
	Agree what to say if someone else answers	
	Check Welcome pack received and understood	
	Confirm whether they want to proceed with approach	
	Agree time for first 'support session' (30 minute window)	
	Check access to a DVD player	
	Check access to broadband internet – and preference for use. Ask to have this switched on if plan to use when you next call	
	Ask to read *Starting out/Write all over* book – and to complete mood scales in advance of appointment if they can	
	Agree you will text to remind of the next appointment time	
	Goodbye – look forward to working with you	

1	**Support session 1: welcome**	
	Text reminder 30 minutes before appointment	
	Introduction reminder – you/them – recheck names to use	
	Do you have a pen and paper?	
	Explain there may be some pauses as you make notes	
	Agree an 'escape' word/phrase if someone comes in and interrupts them (phone only)	
	Discuss briefly their problems – impact on life Point out that ***Understanding why you feel /Why do I feel so bad*** book they have got in their pack will help them find out more about how low/anxious mood is affecting them – and how to change things for the better	
2	**Introduction to the CBT approach**	
	Link this workbook approach with the person's own specific mentioned problems (workbooks and modules will help you tackle the … xxx)	
	Cognitive behavioural therapy – what it means – avoid jargon	
	What you will learn (practical life skills addressing your problems) – a treatment of choice (NICE/national treatment guidelines)	
3	**Clarify choice of resource**	
	Choice of resources to suit how you want to work – key written resources to work through *Many people prefer to see some examples of how other people have used the approach – so we also offer LLTTF DVD or www.livinglifetothefull.com: adds to what you can learn* **If online** talk through a quick overview of the LLTTF site and key features. Sign them up for the reminder newsletters. Show the forum and consider a trial post (hello I'm new)	
4	**Working together with a plan**	
	Describe total number of support sessions/time available (usually 4–6 contacts of up to 2–3 hours)	
	Common and normal to feel demotivated – or to find change difficult to start with	
	Therefore we will work together – regular support/motivate	
	The pack I sent send contains key information sheets (show this if face to face)	
	Make a clear plan for what to do next – using **Planner sheet (introduce) in the Welcome pack**	
5	**Goals**	
	We'll check progress each session using the Review sheets Complete Mood Rating in Welcome pack now	
	Aim is to help you 'turn the corner'	
	If by the end of the support you still feel you need extra support we can discuss that with your GP	

6	**Next steps using the resources – other session(s)**	
	First step is to find out more about why you feel as you do/get started	
	Point to the *Understanding why you feel as you do workbook/Why do I feel so bad book* to be used first	
	Identify key points that resource will cover (i.e. Why do I feel so bad?) – Plus first online module *(Starting out) if they wish/DVD Introduction*	
	Set a clear plan for what to do next (module/book) – using **Planner sheet**	
	Introduce **Review sheet** to structure the discussion for next time. Complete Mood rating scale on the day	
7	**Ending the session**	
	Quick summary recap of key points	
	Confirm a time and number for the next call/contact (30 minute window)	
	Agree you will text to remind of this	
	Agree how much you will chase them if they miss an appointment: it's common when feeling low to talk ourselves out of things – or just forget. You know you – how much would it help for me to really chase you to remind you of appointments?	
	Encourage/praise/motivate. Brief review of what actions agreed to do this week	

Follow-up sessions checklist: reviewing and planning

1	**Welcome back and scene setting**	
	Text reminder 30 minutes before appointment	
	Nice to see/hear you again – we have about x (usually 20) minutes again this session	
	Brief overview of this session (we'll check how your using the approach is going, discuss your mood scores, choose a next target to focus on and then make a plan of how to do that). Is that okay?	
	Doesn't matter if there have been problems/didn't like it – I'm here just to check and help	
	Have you been able to complete the **Review sheet**?	
	Have you been able to complete the **Mood rating**? Go through outcome and record. Respond with team risk response if positive risk item	
2	**Use of the approach this week**	
	Review experience of using/not the materials using the structure on the **Review sheet**	
	Have you used them – if yes – praise If no – look at blocks from **Review sheet** – and problem solve solutions (problems are common – great opportunity to learn)	
	Choose to stick/apply current workbook – or choose to cover new resources/worksheets or modules as needed – and give brief overview/rationale • Good initial topics to focus on are reduced activity/can't be bothered doing anything • Sleep/medication concordance	
	Agree a clear plan for what to do using **Planner sheet**	
3	**Ending the session**	
	Quick summary recap of key points	
	Confirm a time and number for the next call/contact 30 minute window	
	Encourage/praise/motivate and brief review of what actions agreed to do this week	

7 Further information and resources

www.fiveareas.com

This resource has been developed with the intention of providing a useful source of information, practical advice and support for people working using the Five Areas resources. We aim to provide access to high quality and informed content that will be of genuine use to those who access it.

www.livinglifetothefull.com/www.llttf.com

Living Life to the Full is a powerful free life skills resource. The course is designed to supplement and support people using the Overcoming depression and low mood/anxiety books – or the Little CBT Books/DVD.

www.llttfi.com/www.overcomingbulimiaonline.com
www.overcominganorexiaonline.com

Sophisticated computerised CBT package for use with people with problems of depression, bulimia, and for carers and friends of those with anorexia.

www.fiveareasonline.com

Read the Little Books, screen-reader and large print versions.

www.fiveareastraining.com

Practitioner online training modules addressing a wide variety of low intensity support skills both one to one and in classes.

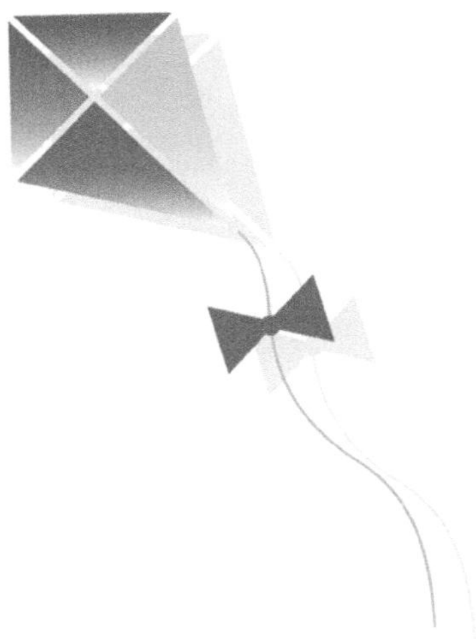

Index

accessibility 9–10
  LLTTF classes 116–20
  training 9
  written resources 129, 137–8
    increasing 140
activity, reduced
  making changes 20, 27
  vicious circle of 20, 46
  see also behaviour
adolescents *see* teenagers
Amazing Bad-Thought-Busting Programme 118
anorexia
  carers 57
  online service 212–13
anxiety
  Big CBT books on 131
    in IAPT service 194–5
    key elements of workbooks 144
    target audience 133
    teenagers 133
  control training (ACT) 156
  in LLTTF classes, your own 121
  progressive exposure and response prevention 4
anxiety disorders, key symptoms 44, 45, 46–52
appointments, missed
  reasons 93–4
  responding to 100–1
Are you strong enough to keep your temper? 136, 137
arthritis 55, 56
assertive follow-up 137
assessment 29–31, 36–77
  10 minute 38–41, 42
  30 minute 41, 42
  60 minute 41–2, 42
  as add-on to usual assessment process 29
  advanced skills 31
  in busy teams and for CPA meetings 30
  carrying out/conduct of 36–7, 63–76
  collaborative 36–77
  common questions 29–30
  first contact, by IAPT team 189–90
  learning and support 136–7
  low intensity CBT 13–17
  patient views 37
  practitioner assessing himself (when moderately upset) 60, 61
  practitioner views 37
  producing your own toolkit 89–90
  purpose/importance 42–3, 70
    informing patient of 64
  structured, informing patient 64
  supervisor 168
assumptions/schemas 24, 25
asynchronous approaches to electronic support 96–8
attitude gains in training, evaluating 177
audio resources
  patient 156
  practitioners
    supervision recording 163–5
    training 176–7
automatic thoughts, negative 17, 24, 25
avoidance
  in health anxiety 50
  in panic disorder 47
  tackling/making changes 21, 27–8
  vicious circle of 21
  see also safety behaviour

BABCP (British Association for Behavioural and Cognitive Psychotherapies) 3, 159, 169
Beck, Aaron 2, 3, 45
behaviour or activity, altered 13, 59
  in 10 minute assessment 39
  asking questions about 67–8
    impact on daily life 74–5
  in Big CBT books 15
  in Little CBT Books 16
  in llttfi.com package 16
  making changes 22, 23, 24–9
  mental health disorders 44
    dementia 54
    depression 44, 47
    flying phobia 52
    generalised anxiety disorder 45, 46
    health anxiety 51
    obsessive compulsive disorder 49

panic disorder 44, 47, 48
paranoid beliefs 53
outcome of guided CBT affected by 81
patterns of 19
helpful 19, 23
repeated 15, 17
physical health disorders 56
practitioner's
in self-assessment 61
in self-reflection 167
in supervision 160, 161
in systemic CBT 32
thoughts and, links 72
vicious circle 22, 46
behavioural activation in depression 4, 19
behavioural experiments for changing beliefs 25–6
beliefs
changing 24–6
paranoid 52–3
bibliotherapy *see* book-based CBT
Big (Large) CBT books 28–9, 131–4
assessment 15
classes based on 124
course 184
high-quality copies 134
linking with other resources 138–9
notes for budget holders and commissioners 140
overview 130, 131–4
problem solving 26
target audience 133
workbooks *see* workbooks
blended learning 130, 138–9
bodily sensations *see* physical symptoms
book-based CBT self-help (bibliotherapy) 6, 39–40
in action
in Canada, with telephone support in depression 192–3
with GP support 190–1
in IAPT service 192–5
schools in Scotland 204–5
social service delivery via telephone and LLTTF classes 197–8
advantages 128–9
assessment in 39–40
disadvantages 14, 129
patients who can't use books 14
see also workbooks
British Association for Behavioural and Cognitive Psychotherapies 3, 159, 169
bulimia, online service 210–11, 233
bulletin boards 97

Canada, five areas book and telephone support 192–3
care programme approach (CPA) meetings, assessment for 30
carers
responses 56–7
support from 99
workbooks for 57, 99
case management 9, 159, 159–60, 162, 163
catastrophising 17, 18
CDs, relaxation 156
change
making 24
in avoidance 21, 27–8
in behaviour 22, 23, 24–9
linking areas to possibility of 72–3
in reduced activity 20, 27
obstacles to 85–6
resources for 28–9
targets *see* targets
chronic fatigue 55
classes and groups 110–25
historical aspects 110–11
LLTTF *see* Living Life to the Full
practical steps in starting and running 112–13
clinical services *see* services
clinical skills supervision 159, 160, 162, 163, 167
collaborative assessment 36–77
collaborative relationship (and working together) 101, 103
face to face support 224, 226
telephone support 228, 230
colour worksheets *see* worksheets
commiseration, remote support 105
'common factors' 43
communication (of CBT to patients)
difficulties 7–8, 14, 62–3
the Five Areas model 17
on avoidance 21
on helpful behaviour 23
on reduced activities 20
on unhelpful behaviour 22

skills *see* competencies and skills
supportive 82
in face to face support 224
in telephone support 228
see also information; language; questions
community settings, five areas in action 197–200
competencies and skills
in assessment, advanced 31
in communication 43
in face to face support 224
in telephone support 228
in supervision delivery 159
in training 170–2
evaluating gains 178
computerised CBT (cCBT) 6, 149
patients unable to do 14
for support 97
see also laptops; online resources
conditional beliefs 24
confidentiality and privacy 64
online data 153
continued professional development (CPD) 173
copying 150
Big CBT books 134
Little CBT books, not allowed 134
LLTTF material 120, 131
courses 9, 178, 181–2
research in 182
see also training
credit card-sized cards accompanying LLTTF DVD 155
criticism of self 18

daily life, exploring impact of problem on 73–6
data protection and privacy issues 153
delivery of CBT
case for 4–6
challenges to 7–9
dementia 54
depression (and low mood) 45–6
behavioural activation 4, 19
Big CBT books on 131, 132, 133
key elements of workbooks 141
teenagers *see* teenagers
with telephone support in Canada 192–3
key symptoms 45–6, 47
postnatal *see* postnatal depression
self-help 4
Depression Alliance Scotland involvement
LLTTF classes
DVD 124
for university students 201
LLTTF free online course 206–7
LLTTFi course 208–9
development of CBT 2–3, 3
diagnosis 43–4
60 minute assessment 38
discharge with self-reviews, preparing for 105–6
disclosure *see* self-disclosure
discussion groups
reflective practice 162
training 173, 180
disorder-specific changes (in different mental health presentations) 44
disruptive person in LLTTF classes 121
distance support *see* telephone support
distress (patient) over assessment 29–30
Doing Well by People with Depression Programme 6
DVDs 149
LLTTF 123, 137, 155

Easy 4 step plan 26, 27, 89, 118
eating disorders, online services 210–13, 233
Edinburgh University students, LLTTF classes 201–2
editable paper resources (LLTTFi) 152
education *see* learning; training
electronic methods *see* email; online resources
email support 96–8
key components 104–5
LLTTF regular reminders 153
questionnaires 100
emotions *see* feelings
encouragement 82
Enjoy your baby 136
events *see* situations
evidence-base for CBT 2, 3
low intensity-working 4
experiments (using) 84
behavioural, for changing beliefs 25–6
exposure (in anxiety), progressive 4

face to face support 93–4, 224–8
key points for checklist 224–8
questionnaires before 100

fainting, phobias 51
fear (being scared)
  attending appointment 93
  of change 85–6
feelings/emotions/moods
  carer's, and overinvolvement 57
  differentiated from thoughts 60–2
  language of 62–3
  outcome of guided CBT affected by 81
feelings/emotions/moods, altered 13, 59
  in 10 minute assessment 39
  asking questions about 66
  in Big CBT books 15
  links
    with physical symptoms 73
    with thoughts 72–3, 73
  in Little CBT Books 16
  in llttfi.com package 16
  mental health disorders 44
    depression 44, 47
    flying phobia 52
    generalised anxiety disorder 44, 46
    health anxiety 51
    obsessive compulsive disorder 48, 49
    panic disorder 44, 48
  patterns 19
    repeated/recurring 17, 19
  physical health disorders 56
  practitioner's
    in self-assessment 61
    in self-reflection 167
    in supervision 160, 161
  in systemic CBT 32
first contact (introduction)
  assessment by IAPT team 189–90
  face to face support 225
  telephone support 229
five areas model
  in action 187–215
  key elements 12–34
flying phobia 52
follow-up
  assertive 137
  checklist
    in face to face support 227
    in telephone support 232
  of missed appointments 101
foreign language, translations 14, 140
forums, online 153–4
friends providing support 99

general practitioner support, five areas books with 190–1
generalised anxiety disorder, key symptoms 44, 45, 46
'Go for It!' slide 122
goals *see* targets
good practice guidelines, audio/video recording 164–5
Google 148
GP support, five areas books with 190–1
ground rules, LLTTF classes 120
groups *see* classes; discussion groups
guided CBT 6–7
  challenges to delivery of 7–9
  competencies for delivery of 170
  factors affecting outcome 80–6
  rating scale in training 178, 179

health *see* mental health disorders; physical health
high intensity CBT 31–3
  assessment 31–3
  case for delivery 4–6
  challenges to delivery 7–9
  expert practitioners' view (compared with low intensity working) 8
  low and, relationship between 101
  training/courses 189
historical development 2–3, 3
  teaching in classes 110–11
How to fix almost everything 135
How to use the Little CBT Books: a practitioner's guide 135
hypochondriasis, key symptoms 50, 51

I can't be bothered doing anything 135
I feel really bad! A guide for turning things around 135
I feel so bad I can't go on 136
IAPT *see* Increasing Access to Psychological Therapies
ice-breakers, LLTTF classes 120
icon-style summary model (llttfi.com package) 16
I'm not good enough: how to overcome low confidence 136
inclusivity, LLTTF classes 116–20
Increasing Access to Psychological Therapies (IAPT) programme 6, 122
  first contact assessment 189–90

Overcoming Anxiety book 194–5
information, patient 7–8
confidentiality *see* confidentiality
see also communication; language; questions
internet *see* online resources
introductory contact *see* first contact

knowledge gains in training, evaluating 177

language 6–7
complexity and difficulties in communication 7–8, 14, 62–3
of emotion 62–3
foreign, translations 14, 140
of physical symptoms 62–3
laptops in training
audio 176–7
presentations 175–6
learning
assessment 136–7
blended 130, 138–9
lifelong, facilitating 166–7
outcome *see* outcome
lecturing style in LLTTF classes, avoiding 121
licence, LLTTF classes 112–13
life *see* daily life; situations
lifelong learning, facilitating 166–7
Little CBT books 28–9, 134–6
in action
housing workers 195–6
schools in Scotland 204–5
social services 197–8
assessment 16
key features 147
linking with other resources 138–9
DVD 138, 155
worksheets 135–6, 138, 155
in LLTTF classes 119, 120, 197–8
notes for budget holders and commissioners 140
overview 130, 134–6
problem solving 26
target audience 134
live (synchronous) electronic support 96
Live longer: have a heart attack 136
Living Life to the Full (LLTTF) 151–4
classes 111–12, 197–8
introducing and supporting 114–20
Little CBT books 119, 120, 197–8
in Northern Ireland 199–200
practical delivery issues 120–3
in Scotland 201–4
in South Tyneside 197
differences from LLTTFi website 149–50
DVD 123, 138, 155
online resources 13, 16, 123, 151–4
in action (Scotland) 206–7
support associations 154
website (lttf.com) 33, 59, 90, 96, 124, 125, 133, 138, 156, 182, 206–7, 233
Living Life to the Full Interactive (LLTTFi) website (llttfi.com) 6, 13, 40, 96, 149–51, 208–9
data protection and privacy 153
differences from LLTTF website 149–50
five areas icon-style summary model 16
key features (patient's perspective) 151
pilot service in Scotland 208–9
LLTTF *see* Living Life to the Full
LLTTFi *see* Living Life to the Full Interactive
locally-delivered training
'selling' the idea 172–3
using practice and review sessions 180
location of classes 116
low intensity CBT
assessment 13–17
case for delivery 4–6
expert practitioners' view (compared with high intensity working) 8
high and, relationship between 101
supervision for 9, 165–6
training 9, 169

mental filter, negative 18
mental health disorders, key symptoms 44, 45–54
mental health primary care team, self-help clinic 214–15
metaphors to describe emotions 62
mind-reading 17, 18
monitoring progress (keeping on track) 139
LLTTF classes 122
mood
altered *see* feelings
low *see* depression
monitoring, LLTTF classes and 122
motivation, aiding/boosting 82, 84
MP3/MP4 files 113, 156
players 149, 156, 163

multimedia resources 148–56
online *see* online resources

National Health Service IT rules and regulations, structured support and 97
national initiatives for locally-delivered training 172
negative automatic thoughts 17, 24, 25
negative mental filter 18
negative predictions 18
newsletters, LLTTF online 153
NHS IT rules and regulations, structured support and 97
Northern Ireland, LLTTF classes 199–200
note-taking in assessment 64

obsessive compulsive disorder, key symptoms 44, 48–9
online resources 151–4, 233
for assessment 13, 16, 39–40
books 138
for support 96–8, 151–2, 183, 206–13, 233
in action 206–13
audio downloads 156
LLTTF *see* Living Life to the Full
questionnaires 100
for training 33, 182, 233
see also computerised CBT
outcome (of learning)
guided CBT, factors affecting 80–6
measuring 122
Overcoming Anorexia Online 212–13, 233
Overcoming anxiety, stress and panic 131, 133
in IAPT service 194–5
key features of workbooks 144
Overcoming Bulimia Online 210–11, 233
Overcoming depression and low mood 131, 132
key elements of workbooks 132, 141, 143
target audience 133
with telephone support in Canada 192–3
Overcoming postnatal depression 131
key features of workbooks 145
Overcoming teenage low mood and depression 131
key features of workbooks 146

pain, long-term 55
panic disorders and panic attacks
Big CBT books on 131
key elements of workbooks 144
target audience 133
teenagers 133
key symptoms 44, 46–7, 48
paper resources (LLTTFi), editable 152
paranoid beliefs 52–3
past events 30
PDF versions of workbooks 5
peer support 99
phobias, specific, key symptoms 51–2, 53
photocopying 140
Big CBT books 134
Little CBT books, not allowed 134
LLTTF material 120, 131, 134
physical health
anxiety, key symptoms 50, 51
disorders of, key symptoms 55
physical symptoms/bodily sensations, altered 13, 59
in 10 minute assessment 39
asking questions about 66
in Big CBT books 15
in Little CBT books 16
in llttfi.com package 16
mental health disorders 44
dementia 54
depression 45, 47
flying phobia 52
generalised anxiety disorder 44, 45, 46
health anxiety 50
obsessive compulsive disorder 49
panic disorder 44, 46, 48
paranoid beliefs 53
outcome of guided CBT affected by 81
patterns of 19
repeated/recurring 17
patterns of emotions and 19
physical health disorders 56
practitioner's
in self-assessment 61
in self-reflection 167
in supervision 160, 161
in systemic CBT 32
thoughts and emotions worsened by 72
physical symptoms/bodily sensations, language of 62–3
pilot interventions 6
Scotland 6, 208–9

using results of 173
Plan, Do, Review approach 86–9, 93, 102
in face to face support 224
in telephone support 228
in training 177
see also review
Planner sheet 76, 86, 87, 88–9, 151, 155, 221
planning in follow-up sessions
face to face support 227
telephone support 232
posters, LLTTF class 115, 116–18
postnatal depression
Big CBT books on 131
workbook 145
colour worksheet 136
Powerpoint 175, 176
practical problems *see* problems
praise, remote support 104–5
predictions, negative 18
preference (of patient) for resource types 129
presentations (for trainees) 175–6
primary care mental health team, self-help clinic 214–15
privacy *see* confidentiality and privacy
problems (practical)
practitioner statement of 38
solving 26–7, 89
resources 28
working between LLTTF sessions on 122
progress, monitoring *see* monitoring
progressive exposure (in anxiety) 4
projectors for presentations 175–6

question(s)
asking by patient before beginning assessment 65
asking the patient 63, 65–70, 73–5
questionnaires when offering 99–100
questionnaires when offering remote support 99–100

rapport 82
readability and reading age 7–8, 130
reassurance 82
Reclaim your life 136
reflective practice/self-reflection 162, 162–3, 166–7, 174
relationships (patient–practitioner) 43, 82
collaborative *see* collaborative relationship
therapeutic *see* therapeutic relationship
relaxation CDs and downloads 156
remote support *see* telephone support
research in training courses 182
resources 219–33
multimedia *see* multimedia resources
packs (for practitioners and patients) 139
problem solving 28
self-help *see* self-help
support *see* support
training 33, 182, 233
responses
carer 56–7
to common problems faced by practitioners 106–7
prevention (in anxiety) 4
review 102
in follow-up sessions
of face to face support 227
of telephone support 232
locally-based sessions 180
Review sheet 86, 88, 89, 123, 151, 155, 222–3
see also self-reviews
role-play (supervisor/supervisee) 163
room layout for LLTTF classes 116

Safe Inside Safe Outside (SISO) 195–6
safety behaviour
health anxiety 50
panic 47
see also avoidance
scary feelings and thought *see* fear
schemas 24, 25
schizophrenia 52–3
schools in Scotland 203–5
Scotland
Depression Alliance in *see* Depression Alliance Scotland
LLTTF online course 206–7
pilot interventions 6, 208–9
schools 203–5
university students 201–2
scripts
class (session) 116
support 103–4, 224–32
secondary schools in Scotland 203–5
self-assessment 13, 39–40
by practitioner (when moderately upset) 60, 61
self-criticism 18

self-disclosure
  LLTTF classes 120–1
  by practitioner, avoiding 105
self-help 6, 6–7
  book-based *see* book-based CBT
  clinic in a primary care mental health team 214–15
  competencies for delivery of 170–2
  depression 4
  resources 24, 31, 39
    design problems 8
    written *see* book-based CBT
self-practice (by practitioner) 162, 167, 174
  assessment (when moderately upset) 60, 61
self-reflection/reflective practice 162, 162–3, 166–7, 174
self-reviews, preparing for discharge with 105–6
sensations, bodily *see* physical symptoms
services, clinical 187–215
  in action 187–215
  discussion groups *see* discussion groups
  patient information on availability 7–8
  supervision incorporated into 158–9
  workforce development needs 173
seven-step plan 26, 27
situations (people and events faced in life) 13, 59
  in 10 minute assessment 39
  asking questions about 66
  in Big CBT books 15
  in llttfi.com package 16
  mental health disorders
    dementia 54
    depression 45, 47
    flying phobia 51
    generalised anxiety disorder 45, 46
    health anxiety 51
    obsessive compulsive disorder 49
    panic disorder 48
    paranoid beliefs 53
  outcome of guided CBT affected by 81
  past 30
  physical health disorder 56
  practitioner's
    in self-assessment 61
    in self-reflection 167
    in supervision 160, 161
  in systemic CBT 32
skills *see* competencies and skills
SMART objectives 89, 90, 93
smoking cessation 136
social services, Little CBT books delivered by 197–8
Starting out 79, 131, 141, 220, 225, 229
step-by-step approach 83–4
  structured support 93
Stop smoking in 5 minutes 136
stress
  Big CBT books on 131
    key elements of workbooks 144
    target audience 133
    teenagers 133
  carer 56
  see also distress
structured assessment, explaining to patient 64
structured practice 174
structured support 92–109
students *see* schools; university students
suicide prevention, book on 136
supervision 158–66
  competencies 159
  incorporation into service 158–9
  for low intensity working 9, 165–6
  models 9, 159–60
  patient use of materials 164
support 92–109
  assessment 136–7
  GP, five areas books with 190–1
  importance 92
  LLTTF in *see* Living Life to the Full
  methods of delivery 93–8
    see also specific methods
  patient information on available options 7–8
  of practitioners 154, 169–85
  practitioners able to provide 98–9
  remote *see* remote support
  resources 96–8, 151–2, 183
    LLTTF 13, 16, 123, 151–4
    questionnaires 100
  scripts 103–4, 224–32
  structured 92–109
  using the right tone to 82
sustainability of locally-delivered training 172
symptoms
  key
    in mental health disorders 44, 45–54

in physical health disorders 55
physical *see* physical symptoms
synchronous approaches to electronic support 96–8
systemic CBT 32

targets and goals (for change)
choosing 24, 64, 82–3
in face to face support 226
identifying key targets 17
setting, in short-/medium-/long-term 84
in telephone support 230
teaching
to groups of patients *see* classes
to practitioners *see* training
technology for training 175–7
teenagers, Big CBT books
on anxiety, stress and panic 133
on low mood and depression 131, 133
key features of workbooks 146
telephone (remote/distance) support 94–6, 228–32
in action 197–8
Canada 192–3
key components 104–5
key points checklist 228–32
online courses and 152
questionnaires 99–100
10 things you can do to make you feel happier straight away 136
text message reminders 95
therapeutic relationship 42, 57, 93, 101, 103, 178
in telephone support 94, 95
Things you do that mess you up 29, 119, 135
thinking/thoughts, altered and unhelpful 13, 59
in 10 minute assessment 39
asking questions about 67
in Big CBT books 15
differentiation from feelings 60–1
links
with behaviour 73
with feelings/emotions 72–3, 73
with physical symptoms 72
in Little CBT Books 16
in llttfi.com package 16
making changes 24–9
mental health disorders 44
dementia 54
depression 44, 45, 47
flying phobia 52
generalised anxiety disorder 44, 45, 46
health anxiety 51
obsessive compulsive disorder 44, 49
panic disorder 44, 48
paranoid beliefs 53
outcome of guided CBT affected by 81
patterns/types/styles 17, 18
repeated 15, 17
physical health disorders 56
posters (for LLTTF classes) 117–18
practitioner's
in self-assessment 61
in self-reflection 167
in supervision 160, 161
see also negative automatic thoughts
thoughts *see* thinking
time issues/considerations
assessment 38–42
informing patient 64
supervision and reflective practice 162–3
support 101–3
training courses 181–2, 184
training 9, 169–85
arranging 183
being effective in
before start of session 174
during session 175
courses *see* courses
format for delivery of 174–6
knowledge and attitudes during, measuring changes in 177–8
locally-delivered, 'selling' the idea 172–3
in low intensity working 9, 169
overcoming common problems 180–1
Plan, Do, Review model in 177
realistic goals 172
relevant/varied/interesting content 173–4
resources 33, 182, 233
skills *see* competencies and skills
views of assessment during 37
translations, foreign language 14, 140
treatment
book resources and 137–8
making links to 75–6
patient presenting with clear focused request for 40–1
supervision of plan and delivery 161
trust 82

university students, LLTTF classes 201–2
unwell person in LLTTF classes 121
usability, resource 130

vicious circles 14, 17, 45, 68, 84
of avoidance 21
Little CBT books 16
in pain (long-term) 55
posters (for LLTTF classes) 117
of reduced activity 20, 46
of unhelpful behaviour 22, 46
video resources
in supervision 163–5
in training 174
virtuous circle 19, 23

warm-ups, LLTTF classes 120
websites *see* online resources
welcoming 220
in face to face support 225
in follow-up sessions 227
in LLTTF classes 116, 120
in telephone support 229, 230
in follow-up sessions 232
well-being, colour worksheets 136
Why do I feel so bad? 135, 225, 226, 229, 230, 231
Why does everything always go wrong? 135
WISH Programme 6, 206–7
workbooks 40, 128, 129, 138, 139
Big CBT Books 131, 147
Overcoming anxiety, stress and panic 144
Overcoming depression and low mood 132, 141, 143
Overcoming postnatal depression 145
Overcoming teenage low mood and depression 146
for carers 57, 99
PDF versions 5
workforce development needs of services 173
working together *see* collaborative relationship
worksheets (incl. coloured versions), linked 118–19, 138
Big CBT books 138
Little CBT books 135–6, 138, 155
online courses 152
workshop, one-day 184
Worry Box: all you need to end anxiety 136
Write all over your bathroom mirror 79, 91, 135, 225, 229
written resources *see* book-based CBT; paper resources

young persons, LLTTF classes 123
see also teenagers